Praise for
Something More Than Love

"If you're looking for an easy read you can leave on your nightstand, this book isn't for you. You will fall in love with this couple and ride out their story with them to the end. *Something More Than Love* may be a memoir, but it reads like a novel, one you will not be able to put down. It's full of suspense, drama, belly laughs, and gut punches. And if you've never wrestled with life's hardest questions (e.g., mortality, the afterlife, God, or final goodbyes), this book also isn't for you. It's a masterclass on what cancer can take from us, but more importantly, what it cannot.

Being that this memoir is such an emotional read, at first you may overlook how much practical information it holds, from being a patient advocate to comforting a grieving widow to the definition of palliative care. This book is a raw look at what the end of life truly looks like and what it means for those of us left behind.

As you read, you may feel surprised that you were able to digest such unfiltered details regarding the dying process. It's truly a roller coaster, and in any other context some of the details would be intolerable. The reason you will continue to hope against hope and take all the harsh realities in stride is simple: At its core, this book is a love story. And if you can't resist a true love story, then this book just may be for you."

~Amanda D'Angelo, PhD (a.k.a. "Mandy")
Clinical Health Psychologist

Something More Than Love

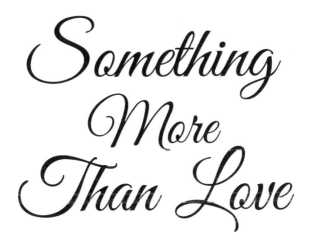

Something More Than Love

*When Your Husband Dies and
Takes Half Your Heart With Him*

PATTY GILBRIDE

Publish Your Purpose
141 Weston Street, #155
Hartford, CT, 06141

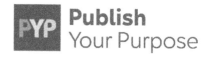

The opinions expressed by the Author are not necessarily those held by Publish Your Purpose.

Ordering Information: Quantity sales and special discounts are available on quantity purchases by corporations, associations, and others. For details, contact the author at thebluebutterflyinme@gmail.com.

Edited by: Nancy Graham-Tillman
Cover design by: Nelly Murariu
Typeset and ebook design by: Amit Dey

ISBN: 979-8-88797-128-5 (hardcover)
ISBN: 979-8-88797-127-8 (paperback)
ISBN: 979-8-88797-129-2 (ebook)

Library of Congress Control Number: 2024915364

First edition, January 2025

For it was not into my ear you whispered, but into my heart.
It was not my lips you kissed, but my soul.

~Judy Garland

Contents

Foreword

One of our great professional privileges is caring for patients. As doctors who treat cancer, we develop relationships with our patients, ones that reach depths that are unique in medicine. These relationships begin at one of the most vulnerable stages of a patient's life (a new or progressing cancer diagnosis) and are punctuated with countless, varying emotions including hope, joy, laughter, fear, and grief. We are fortunate to rejoice in victories, but at times we must also face defeat, times when cancer has "won" and the limits of our therapies have been reached.

Something More Than Love is not about winning or losing. Rather, it tells the story of the amazing David Gilbride. We knew Dave for only a brief time, yet he was so much more than a cancer patient. His infectious smile and quick wit will forever be etched into our memories. You will undoubtedly feel Dave's presence as you read, even if you never had the fortunate opportunity to meet him personally.

As physicians, our focus is often on our patients; unfortunately, their caregivers are often overlooked. Cancer's impact does not stop with the patient. Its ugly tentacles envelop all who are touched by it, even if merely peripherally. While this book shares so much about Dave's life and journey, you will also learn about the extraordinary Patty Gilbride. When we think of Dave and Patty, they represent the most beautiful and inspiring partnership. Dave's gentleness was the perfect balance to Patty's passion. The fierce love and protection that Patty showered upon Dave left us in awe. Will we have the same degree of advocacy if or when we are confronted with a similar illness?

Whether you're a patient, caregiver, provider, or casual reader, we hope this book invigorates you. We are confident it will make you think about caregivers more deeply and recognize the unsung devotion and energy they provide to their loved ones.

Finally, we plead that you support our fight to stop cancer, in whatever capacity you feel is most appropriate.

Dave, you are missed and will forever remain with us. Rest in peace.

Patty, thank you for trusting us and sharing your beautiful story.

~Dr. Siddharth Sheth, Medical Oncology
~Dr. Brian Thorp, Otolaryngology/Head and Neck Surgery
University of North Carolina at Chapel Hill

A Note from the Author

*E*ven if you don't normally read the opening material of a book, I ask that you read this.

You will be joining me in my recollection of the most intense six months of my life. I'll try to be brief here, but that's like asking a turtle to scratch its own back.

As I said, this is my recollection. This memoir is written in journal format, so it's chronological. However, I've inserted flashbacks of my life as they occurred, which are not chronological. I wrote this journal on an almost daily basis and consider it to be extremely accurate; however, perception is different for everyone. It's possible one of the characters in my book may not recollect the events exactly as I describe them. Speaking of characters, some of their names have been changed to protect their privacy, and many have told me they would like their actual name used.

Please do not use any part of this book as a substitute for your own medical care. Although many physicians have teased me that I am an honorary oncologist, nurse, and dietitian, I am not; I have no medical qualifications. But if you garner information from my book that you believe would benefit you or your loved one, please discuss it with your healthcare provider.

I feel I need to also share a trigger warning: This is an extremely intimate look into my life through a very microscopic lens on traumatic events. Sensitive topics discussed include bodily functions, death, OCD, anxiety, and more. If you feel any of these topics are too triggering for your own mental health, please don't read this. Maybe ask someone who knows you and your sensitivities to read it first and then share their reaction with you.

Thank you for allowing me to share my life and my love for my husband with you. Thank you for helping me heal.

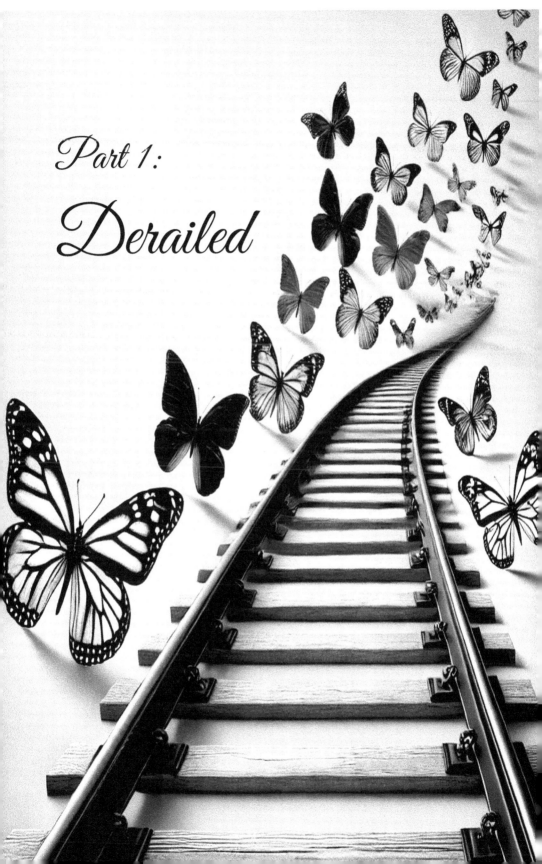

Part 1:

Derailed

Monday, September 18, 2023

For the rest of my life, today will remain one of the most difficult days I have ever experienced.

We spent most of the day anticipating the call. We were still on the fence about getting the feeding tube put in tomorrow. My heart of hearts was telling me we shouldn't do it, but I didn't want to be the one to make that decision. The idea of Dave starving to death makes me sick. I've been so focused on his nutrition since he started having trouble eating over two years ago, how can I watch him starve?

Dave started a new oral chemo regimen, his second, only two months ago, but we don't think it's working. The first chemo pill he took worked great! It kept him stable for over a year. Then the growth around the hole where his nose used to be started. Again. We both knew it was cancer. Again. We prayed it was an infection. But we knew.

When we had it biopsied near the end of July, that day we left for BLT 2023, Dave had developed red bulges outside of his nose hole and on the roof of his mouth. We went anyway because that trip was our second bucket-list trip. Not a true bucket-list trip like the first, but at this point, he's nudging closer to the end of his life's timeline, and we want to do only the things we really want to do and see only the places we really want to see.

While we drove to Virginia—straight from the doctor's office—I kept checking the patient portal for results. By the time Dr. Shilo called and said, "Hi Patty, this is Stu," I knew. My mind raced back to that day in the hospital three years ago when I became Dave's advocate after his first surgery, during the peak of COVID.

Fucking COVID. They won't let me see him in recovery due to new protocols. I'm close to having a tantrum that would put any toddler to shame. Don't you know that's my person! I heard you . . . "He's in recovery" . . . "He's resting peacefully." I need to see him. I NEED to see him.

I'm all prepared to start reciting the patient's bill of rights. As the supervising nurse heads my way, I take a deep breath and try to slow my heart. I'm ready to give her a very hard time. "Mrs. Gilbride, we have a room for your husband. It will just be a bit longer and you can see him on his way to his room," she tells me.

That's when it really starts. That's when I become Dave's advocate. I speak up for Dave, way more than he'd ever speak up for himself. I obsessively check the patient portal, comparing blood work, CT scans, and MRIs. While Dave sleeps, I sit in the chair next to his bed, reading all the radiology reports that come through after the surgery.

I watch the "learning nurse" put a catheter in Dave while the "teaching nurse" observes, and I decide a "learning nurse" will never do one again. I can see the discomfort on Dave's face. I understand this is a teaching hospital, but they won't be learning on my husband.

I will no longer sleep at the hotel. I need to be here. I try to sleep in the chair next to his bed. With all the lights and buzzers and bells, how can anyone actually sleep here?

The nurses are kind to me, but they know I'm watching and listening. I'm sure I've become "that one."

I read additional reports that have come through on the patient portal. I'm panicked to see there are lesions on Dave's lungs. I come to learn they were probably from the bad pneumonia he had when he was seventeen years old, the time he was in the hospital all alone for three months. Not this time. You are not alone this time.

There are three more surgeries after this one, then thirty rounds of radiation, countless infusions of both chemo therapy and immunotherapy, and oral chemo. There's also massage, acupuncture, hyperbaric oxygen therapy, and the special ingredients in Dave's daily dietary shakes. Oh, the shakes! The miraculous shakes. I've consulted with many dietitians regarding these shakes. They get better and better as time goes on, and they change according to Dave's needs. He likes the red ones the most; they look like strawberry but are actually pink because of the beet powder I'm blending in. The doctors and nurses are impressed with the shakes, as are the people in Facebook's Support for People with Oral and Head and Neck Cancer group. Everyone I talk to is impressed with the shakes. It's what I do. Fine-tuning the ingredients in the shakes lets me DO something. I need to keep Dave healthy while he fights this fucking disease. His skin, his nails, his blood, his organs, his bones, his brain, his teeth, his mind . . . all of him must stay healthy while he fights.

And damn, does he fight! Although maybe that's a really poor choice of words. To say Dave "fights" cancer implies that if he dies from cancer, he loses the fight. I'm a bit embarrassed to say that until we encountered cancer, I had no idea how much inner strength my husband had.

Although I suppose that's common. One doesn't know their strength until facing true adversity.

Dave's spirit remains amazing! His will to beat this . . . indescribable! His love for his family is immense! He deals with cancer with more dignity and strength than I ever would have imagined. He does everything the doctors tell him to do, everything I say to do. He doesn't want to let anyone down. Every remedy and concoction I come up with, he tries. He's the perfect patient. And it's during only a few very isolated moments, shared only between a husband and wife, that he shows me his fear and frustration. It never lasts for more than a day or two, and Dave always returns to the strong, optimistic, reliable guy we all count on.

This is how life continues for three years. Dave never actually likes the shakes. He teases me all the time about how awful they are, but he knows they help keep him alive. Eventually, he just can't tolerate them so he starts drinking adult nutrition right out of the bottle. That lasts only for a week or so, then he can't tolerate that. He's having physical difficulties swallowing, and the mental image of these drinks is making him want to barf. We've managed to keep his weight up. I mean, ultimately, he has lost one hundred pounds over the last three years, but in the beginning and up until two weeks ago, he lost slowly. That's when things started taking a turn.

I reach out to Dr. Thorn, our surgeon. He tells us to come in immediately. I love Dr. Thorn. I love Dr. Shilo too. I know they consider us family. When Dave dies—there, I said it— when Dave dies, he won't be a statistic, a number. He will be a person to them. The doctors will probably think of him as an awesome uncle. That's it. Uncle Dave. The great Uncle Dave, much the way he is to his actual nieces and nephews. Dr. Thorn sees us within twenty-four hours and suggests a feeding tube.

When we spoke with Dr. Shilo over the phone, Dave did almost all the talking. It was the first time, really. I, his number-one advocate, took a back seat, and he said what was on his mind: The chemo doesn't appear to be working, the cancer is growing, he's in SO much pain, and we haven't been able to manage it. He thinks it's not just the radiation damage but the cancer that's causing the pain.

If that's the case, what's the sense of the feeding tube? To prolong the pain?

Dave and Dr. Shilo went back and forth conversing, me sitting silently. Definitely a first. Dr. Shilo asked, "Dave, what do *you* want to do?"

And just like that, it was as obvious as a bolt of lightning on a dark night. "I want to stop everything," Dave said.

I knew it was the right thing. I knew that's what Dave truly wanted. Months ago, I told him I would support him 100 percent if we ever got to this point. I asked Dr. Shilo how much time Dave had, though I know doctors don't like to talk numbers when it comes to life expectancy. Dr. Shilo has always avoided it, so I've never asked. But today, I asked him if Dave had a month. Dr. Shilo said weeks, which to me meant only two to three.

As I sat on the kitchen stool next to Dave at the dining table, I felt my heart tumble right out of my chest, bounce off my knees, and hit the floor with a hard thud.

Dave, then we, decided to stop the chemo pills, cancel the feeding tube, and switch from palliative care to hospice. When we got off the phone, I cried. I wailed. I crawled off the kitchen stool and into Dave's lap, just like I did in Dr. Thorn's office during the early days of the cancer train.

Dave is in the examining chair; I'm sitting across from him. Dr. Thorn has bad news for us. He tells us the cancer is aggressively growing. When Dave was first diagnosed, we were told we had an 85 percent chance of being cancer-free for five years with the protocol we were following. So much for five years . . . it's been only six months, and the cancer is growing.

Dr. Thorn leaves the room. Dave keeps his composure. I lose it. I crawl into his lap and cry. Oh God, do I cry. I'm not ready to lose him. Dave comforts me. "It's okay," he says, "I'm not going anywhere just yet."

Dave says those words to me whenever he sees me crumble. "I'm not going anywhere . . . just yet" are words of comfort. They're the words that bring me back from a puddle of mush to a fighting-strong, number-one advocate. Somehow I believe that when he says them, they must be true. Dave's words have that effect on me.

But now? Now everything is about managing Dave's pain. It was so clear after he made the decision to stop all treatment that it was the right one for him. He felt solid. He felt . . . relief. No more suffering, no more disfigurement, no more treatment. So, I called the nurse practitioner at the palliative care center and told her we were stopping the chemo pills.

Wait . . . that's not quite right.

Since I'm an only child, I'm used to everything always being "I." And well into our marriage, it was *my* house, *my* dog, *my* beach condo, *my* kitchen, *my* future. But during this cancer battle, "I" has become "WE." A big, ginormous, capital WE. WE change the shakes, WE aren't feeling well, OUR blood pressure is a little high, WE need you to do this, WE want that. Somewhere during the last twenty-one years, and after many years of marriage, I've finally become a WE.

So *we* switched over to hospice.

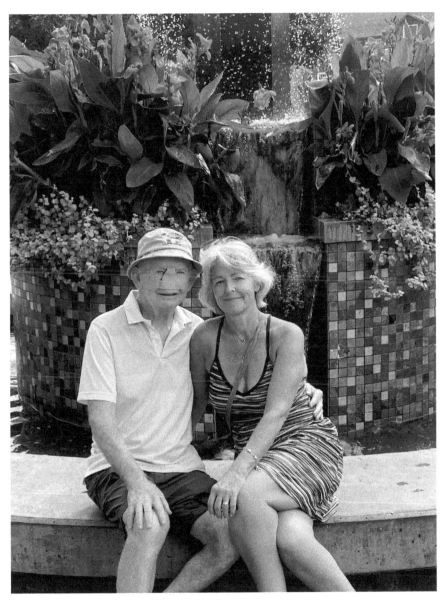

August 9, 2023: Frankenmuth, Michigan, soon after
the start of BLT 2023

Tuesday, September 19

A woman named Shirelle came to the house. When she arrived, I went downstairs to see if she needed help carrying anything. I was halfway down when I first laid eyes on her. She was about my age, maybe a few years older, and had very short gray hair. She looked up and saw me.

In a beautiful accent, she said, "Hello. Are you okay?"

I shook my head no, then burst into tears. I walked down the stairs and fell into her arms.

"Oh, dear, dear, this is so unfair," she said.

Even the hospice nurse knows this is unfair. I liked her immediately. Something about her made me think of Mary Poppins. She's from Zimbabwe. I told her she'll love Dave. I told her EVERYONE loves Dave.

Shirelle made us laugh. When she saw that Dave had a sense of humor, she told us her "boob story." I think she was inspired because Dave asked if there were any nurses who resembled Victoria's Secret models. That's my Dave. Always with a joke.

She prepared us for what hospice entails. Sometimes the information seemed so fact-based; sterile, medical. That's the stuff I'm good at, the stuff I've been handling for the last three years, along with the insurance, the appointments, the patient portal messaging, and all the normal household stuff. Yes, the sterile business stuff I was good at. Then she'd touch on something like a DNR order. Sheesh. Not so sterile anymore.

Shirelle finally called the hospice doctor. Officially, they needed a doctor to do the intake. She sat at our dining table and went through the particulars. "I have David Gilbride here . . . a seventy-year-old man . . ." blah blah blah.

I could hear the doctor on the other end of the phone who was saying yes to some things and no to others. Then he said, "Does he have a big hole in his face?"

You've got to be kidding me! What is he, a fucking frat boy?

Shirelle knew I heard. She kept talking like a pro. When she got off the phone, I repeated his words. She apologized for his insensitivity. Asshole.

I was disappointed to find out that Shirelle would only be our nurse navigator who handled intake, not our hospice nurse. She told us our hospice nurse would reach out in a day and a social worker would contact us to sign the DNR.

Can we stop talking about the DNR? I've done everything I can to keep this man alive for the last three years. CAN WE STOP TALKING ABOUT HOW WE WILL NOT RESUSCITATE HIM?!

Wednesday, September 20

I went out to run some errands today and took Sadie to the woods for some exercise. Myra called. She will be our nurse. It was so nerve-racking waiting to meet the person who will help usher Dave from this life . . . the person who will try to keep him pain-free . . . the person who must be on her A-game.

I'm still his person. I'm still his advocate. Myra, I may be a puddle of mush, crying all the time and heaving sometimes, but you better be good. You need to be better than good. You need to be the best!

Myra arrived on time. She was younger than I would have liked. We sat in the living room and just talked about stuff: her kids—she has one with autism—the ever-growing area, issues with infrastructure . . . blah blah blah. Dave, the most engaging conversationalist I've ever known, was his usual charming self. Even though he's on fentanyl patches and morphine, he's still alert and incredibly likable. I was somewhat standoffish. Under the circumstances, typical me. Myra couldn't have recognized this, but I was surveying her, interviewing her in a way. I'm skeptical about everything.

At some point, I got a phone call. It was the social worker from hospice, the one who will be bringing the DNR paperwork, the one who will be getting Dave to sign a piece of paper saying it's ok to not try to start his heart back up. I could do that myself. I know what Dave wants. Shirelle said that legally, if Dave's heart stops and there's no DNR, I would have to call 911 and the first responders would be obligated to try to bring him back to life, no doubt crushing many of his fragile ribs. That would never happen. As long as Dave wasn't gasping for air, I wouldn't call 911 until I knew he was dead. But I'll play by the rules. I like rules. Now it won't be an issue. With a DNR, I'm supposed to call hospice. They call the funeral home. How nice and neat.

Myra, Dave, and I went about chatting. No tears from me. I was still judging whether Myra was going to be the one. Will she be able to take care of Dave . . . and me? I told her I picked up the five-pack of meds she'd ordered from the drugstore. Hospice calls them "comfort meds" and orders them to be on hand in the house. She said she knew I'd probably already looked at their descriptions. She has a good read on me already. Of course I looked at them. And of course I got upset when I saw drugs for "agitation." Ugh. This is going to be so awful.

When Myra read through the names of each drug and its purpose, I welled up. While my eyes pooled, hers became kind. Really. As she looked back and forth at me and Dave—mostly at me since Dave will probably be unaware at the time these drugs will be used—her eyes softened. They said, "I'm sorry this is happening to you. I know this is so hard. I know you love him. I know you are in so much pain right now."

I wrote a letter to the physician who made that insensitive comment about the hole in Dave's face. Dave calls it a "Patty letter." It's a letter telling the physician how the lack of respect he showed for my husband and his body is completely unacceptable and will not be tolerated; he needs to do better. He *will* do better if he's going to be my husband's doctor for the rest of his life. So when Dave asked Myra whether she sees this doctor at the facility, I knew what he was getting at.

I told Myra that I'd overheard something the doctor said to the other nurse on the phone that was very inappropriate and that I'd written him a letter telling him so. She told me he was thirty-six and needed to be taken down a peg and said she would gladly deliver my letter.

Myra passed the test. I'm still a touch guarded, and we've met her only once, but she passed and is welcome back.

Thursday, September 21

Today a social worker arrived to obtain lots of info from us. His job is to help us with resources, like the VA, financial aid, and a spiritual advisor. But we don't need any resources. His real job was to explain the DNR and get it signed. I saw the yellow piece of paper lying face down on the table and knew what it was.

Isn't it funny that it was yellow? Yellow has been coming up a lot. It started last week when Dave's sister thought the house they were renting across the street from us was yellow when it was actually white with green shutters. All weekend we teased Margaret about the "yellow house" and her blunder. Then, when I was looking online for a dress for Dave's funeral—Ugh. A dress for my husband's funeral—a yellow one popped up. I don't look good in yellow. But I thought about the yellow house. Then there was something else in yellow and now THE piece of paper was yellow.

The social worker waited until the very end of the conversation to present it. He's a really sweet guy, a father of four, and he was going to be a state trooper. Since I retired from law enforcement after twenty-five years, I felt confident telling him he was much better suited for this job. He seemed to appreciate that. Why waste all that compassion?

He flipped over the paper and asked Dave if he knew what it was and understood it. Then he asked me. I shook my head. I couldn't speak. I just kept nodding.

"Does it have to go on the refrigerator?" I squeaked.

"No, it doesn't," he said.

Dave piped up. "But it's in the event she's not here . . . so they know . . ."

Yes. So they know, I thought. *So they know not to break his fragile ribs and pump him full of adrenaline. How awful would that be? To bring him back from death to near death, and for what?*

I put the yellow piece of paper on the fridge—face down. I'll flip it face up when I leave the house, and I'll only leave Dave alone with special people; people I can trust. But in case they forget that they shouldn't call 911 and accidentally do, that yellow piece of paper has to be visible.

The yellow reminds me of that ceramic sun Dave bought me for a garden ornament when we were at the craft show in Poplar Grove. He was often clueless about what to get the girl who has everything, but I found this adorable garden ornament—a yellow, ceramic sun—that had not only a smiley face but a smiley face with personality and character, one I would have loved to put in my garden. I told my friend to make sure Dave knew I wanted that sun for the next gift-giving occasion. She told him, Dave snuck it in the car, and voilà! There it was at the next gift-giving occasion.

Just before I lost myself in that memory, the social worker asked if we'd met Myra yet. We told him we had and that she'd be back in a few days. Then he told me she had a personal issue that would take her away from her job for the whole month of October.

What?! For real? Don't you think that's a critical time to send us a replacement? Someone new to bond with? First

Shirelle, then Myra, then whoever. Well, if someone else comes in October, Myra is done. No offense Myra, but I'm not building a rapport with someone only to have them leave.

At this moment, Forrest Gump enters my mind . . . that's all I have to say about that.

Saturday, September 23

I made blueberry muffins last night using Dave's mom's recipe. I have my own recipe I prefer, one of the recipes that has given me notoriety as a baker. Funny how I decided to make Flo's. They're very simple and made in one bowl. I put my own spin on it, adding a little confectioners' sugar drizzle on the top, though she would have thought they were fine the way they were. I wonder if anyone is thinking, *Look, Patty's fine. She's handling this well; she's baking!* Pfftt. They came out yummy. I wish Dave could taste them.

I've always loved cooking for Dave. Cooking and baking . . . two different skills. I remember the first dinner I made for him. It was that recipe for pork chops with the bone-in, sautéed in a pan with gravy. There were a few peppers and onions sprinkled in too. That recipe has been in my cookbook for over twenty years. Many times I've thought, *Do I really need a recipe to sauté pork chops in a pan?* But every time I flip through my cookbook and see that recipe, I always think about how that first dinner brought a smile to Dave's face. He really enjoyed it!

I didn't know at the time that any meat and gravy meal would be a score with him! I also didn't know that Dave would never, *ever* complain about anything I would make. I think he feels that if I take the time to cook for him, he should eat and not complain. So, I had to determine a way to decide whether a new recipe was really good. That's when we discovered the term "keeper." Instead of asking Dave whether he liked a new recipe, I'd ask him if it was a keeper, a recipe I was supposed to keep and make again. He's always teased that I make so many new recipes he never sees the keepers again. "But if I tell you it's a keeper," he jests, "I'll never see it again."

Sunday, September 24

We had a bit of a rough start this morning. What's unusual is that I was still in bed sleeping with Dave when he woke up. He was alarmed about something and woke me. I was dreaming about puppies. In my dream, a white puppy with brown blotches and a pink nose sat on my shoulder, snuggled under my chin. I woke to the reality of my life. It was a rough way to start the day.

Many hours later, Dave took a nap on the couch with his head on my lap. I stroked his head and he fell asleep easily. I was basically trapped in this position for nearly two hours . . . not wanting to move . . . not wanting to wake him. My eyes drifted around the room. They landed on that beautiful, framed, black-and-white photo of our wedding. Our first dance. In that photo, the pure happiness and love on our faces is obvious. But does anyone really understand the commitment that comes with that day?

The funny thing about that dance is, I'd made Dave take dance lessons with me beforehand. We wanted to do a nice waltz . . . maybe a foxtrot. Well, I didn't know the names of those dances until about fifteen years later, but that's what I'd been envisioning.

The odd part is that when I was young, I said I wanted to have "Can't Help Falling in Love" by Elvis Presley at my wedding; it's the only wedding detail I ever gave any thought to. But you know what? I forgot about it! How does someone forget the song they want at their wedding?

We still can't decide on our song. I suggest "I'll Always Love You" by Taylor Dayne, a popular song.

"No Taylor Dayne," says Dave.

Really? You couldn't care less about music. Why do you care about the dance song at the wedding?

No Taylor Dayne.

We start taking dance lessons and rehearsing to "Unforgettable" by Natalie Cole. I'm doing great at the lessons. Dave . . . well . . . Dave has the rhythm of a White boy.

Midway through the lessons, we change our song. Okay, I change our song. I can't believe we can't have the Taylor Dayne song. I don't think in twenty-one years of marriage he's ever said no to anything I've wanted. I decide the song we'll dance to will be "From This Moment On" by Shania Twain. The words . . . just the perfect wedding song . . .

The big day is finally here. The wedding is beautiful. The weather is beautiful. I've never been happier.

We do the photos and the cocktail hour . . . now it's time for the entrance and the first dance. Our deejay commands, "Please stand up and show some love for Mr. and Mrs. Gilbride."

The music starts, Dave and I sashay into the room, our family and friends applaud, we look into each other's eyes, and . . . I freeze up like my feet are stuck in mud. Can't remember a damn thing! Can't remember the steps! Dave saves the day, leads me around the floor like a pro, and even slips in an unplanned twirl.

I haven't lived that down for twenty-one years.

As Dave woke up and began moving about the house, I told him about my walk down memory lane and asked him whether he thought the Taylor Dayne song was the only time he said no to me in our marriage.

"I think you're right," he said. "And it's a good thing we didn't have that Taylor Dayne song or we never would've lasted this long."

Dave. My funny Dave.

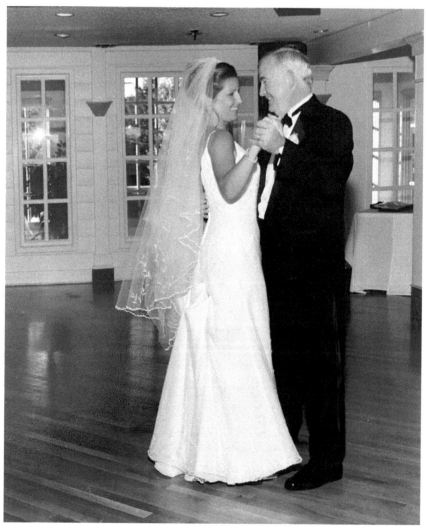

September 7, 2002: First dance at our wedding

Tuesday, September 26

I slept terribly last night. Not like I was crying all night like some nights. I just kept waking up. I knew when I woke at 4:50 a.m. that would be the end of sleeping. I moved closer to Dave in our king-size bed. He takes up so much less space now that he's down one hundred pounds. When I lay my arm around his waist, I can feel that there's no meat on him; his ribs protrude.

At half past five I heard Sadie get up and move to another room. Then I heard her starting to vomit. Great. She went to her favorite carpet to puke. I got up, shuffled her outside to the back deck, then started cleaning the mess and making coffee. About forty-five minutes later, I heard her barking. It was too early for a barking dog, so I slipped outside to investigate the cause of her noise. It was dark and humid. The birds were starting to chirp. It brought me back to when Dave and I spent that week in Lanai, Hawaii, before we started dating.

When we first arrive at our room, I see there is ONE king-size bed. Uh oh. This could be uncomfortable. I thought we'd have separate beds. When we go to bed that night, Dave is a gentleman. Dave is always a gentleman.

He snores so loudly I move from the bed to the deck to the bathtub. When I tell him the next day how disturbing his snoring was, he spends the rest of the week sleeping on the deck. He says that he sleeps better out there. It has a nice lounge chair with a five-inch cushion, and the sound of the waves crashing on the rocks all night makes for a better night's sleep. But the real reason he sleeps so soundly? He knows I'm happy and getting a good night's sleep.

Our body clocks are all thrown off by the time difference, so we wake when it's still dark. But being that we're at a fancy hotel on a trip hosted by a big oil company, they accommodate their guests at all times. We rise for the day, me climbing out of bed and Dave from his lounge chair, at some crazy early time, I don't remember how early . . . probably in the 4–5 a.m. hour.

There's a coffee station down the hall. We leave our room and walk down the hall to this sort of indoor/outdoor paradise. It has furniture and a roof, but it's outdoors. The birds are chirping, and all the vegetation is thriving in the humidity of the morning air before the sun rises.

Dave and I head over to the prepared table that has quite a variety of coffee, tea, and treats. We sit and chat. We don't have the closeness yet for deep talks, but we chat. And boy, does Dave learn how I can chat for hours! And I learn how Dave can listen for hours.

This morning, when I walked outside, it felt just like that morning in Lanai: birds chirping, sun getting ready to rise, humidity in the air. Deep breath. Savor the moment. Savor the memory.

3

Wednesday, September 27

*I*t was five weeks ago tomorrow that we returned home from our thirty-day RV trip. It was a good trip, but it wasn't like last year's. Last year's trip was more of a bucket list trip. It was awesome and perfect! Even all the crap that went wrong was perfect! This trip was a slightly slower pace. Niagara Falls . . . visit family and friends . . . eleven nights in Michigan. Boy, did we love Michigan! Gorgeous lakes, cool August temperatures, and lots of great rail trails for bike riding. Dave uses his e-bike these days, but he's still pretty amazing; we did three twenty-mile rides and several smaller ones.

I haven't taken the bike out since I've been home . . . until yesterday. Yesterday I took Sadie for a longer walk than usual, then went for a bike ride in the afternoon. I wasn't into bike riding when I was in my twenties and thirties. I guess I liked it when I was a kid. I do remember riding bikes with my dad, but the last time I owned a bike I was probably a teen.

When Dave and I were dating he bought me a bicycle. I suppose it was a mountain bike. I think this was probably before they had "hybrids," or good-for-everything bikes. The gears were on the handlebars, and you'd twist the grip to change them. I didn't understand anything about gears, but I lived in a fairly hilly area at the time, so gears were crucial! Dave, always riding behind me, would shout out in an attempt to explain the concept of pulleys to help me grasp the gear system. I'd yell back, "What number should I use . . . on the left or the right?" I like concrete, factual information. I had so much to learn about cycling.

We occasionally took the bikes to Central Park in New York City or on a rail trail in the country. For the life of me, I could not understand why he enjoyed this. But I always enjoyed being outside and was more of an outdoorsy type than Dave, so it was a fair compromise to be outside doing an activity he enjoyed.

After Dave and I got married, we purchased our little one-bedroom condo at the Jersey Shore. Some of our happiest memories occurred there! We brought our bikes to our new place and stuck them in the shed. We went to our little "happy place" pretty much every weekend year-round. In early spring, I realized there wasn't much to do in April at the shore. It was too cold to go to the beach and too nice to sit inside. Dave and I started "tooling around" on the bikes, and we rode around the quiet streets of Spring Lake.

Being a fairly competitive person, one who's never had any sports skills, I wanted to ride further than the last ride. I remember that one day when Dave wasn't at the shore with me, and I decided I was going to ride fifteen miles, then turn around and ride back. Regardless of what happened along the way, I was going to ride a mountain bike thirty miles in total. I can be like that sometimes. Stubborn. I set a goal, and regardless of what happens, I will finish. Sometimes that can be described as grit, sometimes stupidity. But that day I did it. Wait . . . what? I rode thirty miles on my bike! I did it!

My rides with Dave became longer and more interesting after that. Dave joked that all he got to see was my "lovely bum," which he never complained about. I started thinking I might actually be good at this!

I liked to ride just for the sake of riding, to go further and faster than the last time. Dave liked to ride to look at the scenery—whether that was bikinis or buildings. So we had our "together rides," and I had my "Patty rides."

The best way to get Dave to keep riding was to dangle the promise of treats in front of his nose. We would ride fifty miles along the New Jersey coast in a day, stopping for drinks along the way, sticky buns at Park Bakery in Seaside Park, and possibly even ice cream at one of the many ice cream joints that dotted the Jersey Shore. Our bike rides became one of the best things we could share, even though we did them a little differently.

Eventually, I bought that Trek hybrid and we entered organized rides. Those rides had food and drink stations along the way and were usually about thirty-miles in total, with lots of hills and scenery. Dave would give me a kiss and tell me to have fun as he caught a glimpse of my bum pedaling away with the pack. Dave rode at his own pace. He smelled the roses along the way. By the time he'd get to the finish line, I'd usually have my bike packed up and be ready to go. But we would both chime, "Are we ready to eat? Where do we want to get food?" Rides like those worked up such an appetite, and we both loved to eat!

When we retired to the beach in North Carolina, we would ride our bikes to a coffee shop about ten miles away, drink coffee, then ride home. I'd research rail trails in our new state and we would toss the bikes on the back of the car and make it a road trip, always looking for great food and treats along the way. Dave loved to eat! He really loved to eat!

I joined a cycle club for a while so I could keep moving at my pace, but I always enjoyed my rides with Dave. He rode at the same pace. He was predictable and constant. I always knew where he was. That's pretty much how we've lived our lives together: He's predictable and constant, always there.

Anyway, apparently Dave has noticed that I've pretty much stopped all recreational activity. My usual schedule of three days a week at the gym including personal training has stopped. My one day a week with the horses including a riding lesson has stopped. It all stopped when we got home from the trip and Dave took a turn. I thought he just "got sick." I didn't know this was a direct path to the final destination.

Two days ago, Dave heard me planning virtual doctor visits for myself and rearranging my schedule. I'm willing to leave the house only when someone trustworthy is here, and even then it's just for local trips. But Myra came today. The three of us had a very difficult conversation regarding some worst-case scenarios, which made Dave and I tense. Dave addressed me as soon as Myra stepped out of the room to take a phone call.

"You gotta stop," Dave growled, clearly spoken in his annoyed voice.

I didn't say anything. I was angry and sad and thought, *I don't have to stop anything, dammit.*

Myra came back into the room just then, but I knew when she left for the day that Dave and I needed to finish our conversation. Eventually we did.

"What do you mean?" I asked him.

"Well, you're here all the time, and you've stopped doing everything you enjoy. You can't stop living," he said.

"Don't you realize that now that I see how finite your time is, I want to spend every moment with you? I want to absorb you," I retorted.

"I understand that. But you gotta get out. Maybe I want to be alone for fifteen minutes."

"But what if you have a heart attack when I'm not here? I don't want you to die alone."

Dave got the final word: "It's okay. It doesn't matter. I'll be fine. Besides, I'm not having a heart attack today."

How I wish he would have said, "It's okay. I'm not going anywhere just yet," like he's said before. But he didn't.

4

Thursday, September 28

For many, many months, in the back of my mind, I have thought about the fact I will need to buy a dress for Dave's funeral. I haven't dwelled on it, but, living at the beach and having an active casual lifestyle with only occasional dressy events, I really don't have anything suitable for my husband's funeral. I mentioned this to Dave. Yup, I sure did.

Mr. Constant-and-Always-Able-to-Help-Me-Get-Through-Anything suggested I get a "comfortable Hawaiian jumper." Really? Of course he meant it. He didn't know exactly what a jumper was, but I understood his point.

I've started searching online and have an idea of what I might be looking for. I don't want to go to the store for this dress. The whole idea of heading out to shop for a dress for my husband's funeral is such a weighty thought. I've picked out a dress, ordered two sizes, and am waiting for Amazon to deliver. The dress reminds me of Ginger.

People joke that I'm part dog, a dog whisperer, a wannabe dog . . . I just love dogs. When Dave came into my life, he discovered that part of me. My life is not complete without a dog in my home. They are my family members. Dave has always said, "When I die, I want to come back as one of Patty's dogs."

For most of my adult life, I've had two dogs at a time, and they've all been rescues. The deaths of my dogs have been my most painful experiences to date. I've been present for all their euthanasias, except for Gus's, getting down on the floor and holding them in my arms, telling them how much I love them. The moment they cross from life to death has always been particularly difficult for me.

Alive . . . dead.

Here . . . not here.

I just can't grasp it.

My sobs turn to painful, hard crying at these moments of permanent transition. My veterinarians have even cried when they've seen my reaction. Dave has always been there to comfort me during these times.

I remember I was on vacation with my girlfriend when it was time for Gus—Gussie Bear—to cross over. Dave took him to the vet by himself. He told me when I returned home how much harder it was to be the "primary griever." I've been the primary griever for all the others. I've been the one on the floor. I've been the one saying, "It will be okay . . . I love you . . . I love you . . . I love you." I've been the one who's fallen into Dave's arms and bawled like a baby afterward. For Gus, Dave was there alone. I'm sure that was hard on him.

After each of these experiences, I often swear I will never get another dog; I never want to love like that again or hurt like that again. Dave consoles me. He knows in about six months I'll start scrolling through the shelter websites to find our next pup. It could be any gender, any color, any breed, and any age. Several weeks later, he'll see me heading out the door. "I'm going to look at a dog," I'll say. Upon my return, he'll ask, "Did we find a dog?"

I tell him about Esther. Well, that's what the shelter calls her. She's a dumped dog. They named her Esther because she was found around Easter. She's a Wheaton Terrier with a bunch of other stuff mixed in, about seventy-five chunky pounds, and probably has only a few good years left in her. I bring her home for a trial weekend to see how she'll fit into our lives and how Daisy—who'd rather be an only dog—will tolerate her.

We bring her out to the woods on a hike to see if we can decipher her true personality. She isn't the most adventurous, but she wanders around. We return home, and Dave plops on the floor to read the Sunday paper. Esther plops down beside him. Eventually I peek into the living room to see Dave sound asleep on the floor. He and Esther are lying back-to-back, both sleeping peacefully. A bonding moment. Clearly, this dog needs to be part of our family.

I tell the shelter we want her. She certainly doesn't recognize the name the shelter has given her, so I decide to rename her. She reminds me of the dog on the box of Ginger Snaps, so we name her Ginger.

She's so chunky. I put her on a diet by swapping some of her food for canned green beans, something I've done with all my overweight shelter dogs. We take ten pounds off her! The green beans are soon dubbed "Gingey beans." Of course, that becomes a new nickname for Ginger. She will forever be lovingly called Gingey Bean.

That dog makes Dave laugh more than any other dog we've had—nine in total! When Dave comes home from work, I urge Ginger, "Daddy's home! Go say hi to Daddy" as I nudge her out the front door. She walks to the edge of the porch, sees him, and turns around ready to come back inside. Dave always jokes that Ginger is thinking, "Oh, that asshole. Okay, I see him. Can I come back inside now?" It happens day after day and is funny as hell!

One day Ginger is having trouble getting up. She's clearly in distress and panting. We rush her to the emergency vet and they "tap her like a keg." She has fluid around her lungs, probably due to cancer. We're able to take her home, but we're advised that this will happen again. The vet tells us we can tap her again, if we want. Ugh.

For the next month, Ginger's already improved life becomes the life of a queen. She gets scrambled eggs for breakfast and regular trips to the lake where we lie on a blanket and watch the ducks. We're on notice that her life will soon be over. I want to make her happy and absorb as much of her as I can.

About a month after that first incident with the fluid around her lungs, Ginger has a seizure. It's right at bed-time and it's awful! It probably lasts less than a minute, but it feels like it goes on for ten. I say to Dave, "That's it. We're not putting her through this again. I'll make the appointment."

As with all the dogs before her and all the dogs after, it's an awful, heart-wrenching experience. The final goodbye. I know this one will cut Dave deep. She was his "spirit dog." Ever since she plopped on the floor next to him, we knew this was not going to be an obedient dog I trained like all the others. This was going to be a dog that just . . . was.

That weekend, after we euthanize Ginger, we go to our happy place at the beach with just one dog, Daisy. While outside we see a butterfly. I don't know who says it first, but we call out, "Gingey Bean!" From that day forward, every butterfly we see, we cry out, "Gingeyyyy Beannnn!"

So anyway, the dresses came in the mail yesterday. I tried them on alone. I decided I liked it enough to get Dave's opinion. It's not the typical tailored black dress a grieving widow would wear, but it's probably a very typical dress for a grieving

Patty. I slipped into our walk-in closet as Dave got ready for bed, then came out with the dress on, saying, "I don't even know if it's appropriate to ask you this, and I don't know if the dress is appropriate. Do you like this? Is it okay?"

He squinted. His eyes have been failing him lately. "You look great!" he said. "But I'm the wrong person to ask. You always look great to me."

"But do you think it's appropriate? The color and all? I don't think it's common for women to wear off-white to their husband's funeral. Do you see what's all over the dress and understand the significance?" I asked.

"They're butterflies," he said, "and they remind me of Gingey Bean."

I will wear an off-white dress covered with red, blue, and black butterflies to Dave's funeral. I still can't wrap my head around the fact that this will be in my immediate future and he won't be here anymore.

5

Friday, September 29

*J*ames has been here since Monday and is staying until the end of the week. He told me he has some things he needs to talk to his dad about and would like me to be present. James was about twenty-two years old when I married his father, so he was long out of the house and absorbed in his own life as any twenty-two-year-old would be. Even though I've been a part of this family for a long time, James warmed my heart saying he wanted me near when he talked to his dad.

I suspected the things he wanted to talk to Dave about were father-son issues that happened long before I ever came into the picture. James is a psychologist, so he's a trained professional in matters of the mind, yet I know this is extremely difficult for him.

I took advantage of James being around to keep an eye on things, and I got out of the house for a bit. Plus it gave him and his dad some alone time.

James will be leaving tomorrow to drive home to Florida. He still hasn't spoken the words that I know are weighing heavily on his heart. He asked me this morning what was on the schedule for the day. We've had visitors in and out of the house for days. Everyone goes on my calendar and gets a time limit, except Colonel Tom. Colonel Tom is Dave's best friend and can spend as much time with Dave as he wants. It's good for both their souls.

I ran through the schedule for the day with James, and he said today was the day he needed to talk to us. He knows he's running out of time, and this was a conversation that needed to be had in person. I told him I'd make sure it happened this morning. Privately, I told Dave. Dave knows his son's heart and mind need to be set free, and he will do whatever is necessary.

The three of us sat in the living room, Dave in that pink chair where he's usually seated for visitors. Besides the fact this chair is a gorgeous hot pink, it has a firm back and arms, which make it particularly comfortable. But its real advantage is that the front two legs have casters, making it easy to spin in different directions. James sat on the sectional sofa facing Dave, and I sat adjacent to the two of them. We were somewhat in a triangle, with me being in a position to watch as if I were watching a tennis match.

James opened with saying he has wanted to write his dad a letter, but "Saying what I have to say in a letter is like trying to put the wind in a paper bag." I don't know whether he just made that up or he worked on that opening, but it was absolutely perfect for what was about to follow.

I will never divulge the contents of the emotional scene that unfolded today. James was wrought with physical emotion; Dave was the father he's always been . . . like a lighthouse on a stormy night . . . constant . . . reliable . . . sturdy. When Dave saw his son struggling with the emotion that was spilling out of him, he rose from the pink chair and moved towards James, saying, "Come here, Baby J." No doubt Dave has been calling James "Baby J" long before I ever entered their lives.

As an observer, this was the most poignant moment, to date, I have ever witnessed between a father and son. I struggled to fight back tears as Dave and James embraced. It was a moment I will never forget.

6

Sunday, October 1

*L*ast night, as I sat on the couch and Dave rummaged around his briefcase on the dining table, I said to him, "You've taken care of me for twenty-one years." He looked up and, without missing a beat, replied, "Baby, it's the other way around. You've taken care of me."

Wanting to be close to him, I suggested we take a tub together. I imagine most people would phrase that by saying they took a "bath" together. We've taken more tubs in the last six months than we have in twenty-one years of marriage. Dave loves the hot water, especially now that he's cold all the time.

I tossed all my good-smelling stuff into the tub as the water filled the jacuzzi. Rather ironic since Dave doesn't have the ability to smell anything. It's a large tub, and the fifty-gallon water heater is barely sufficient.

With ambient lighting and candles flickering, I slipped into the tub, the overflow drain pressed against my back. When I tub alone, I sit on the other side, the more comfortable way, with my back against the smooth porcelain. But when tubbing with Dave, I don't want him to deal with the discomfort of all the plumbing.

Dave stuck his head through the open bathroom door and said, "You're in already!" as if he was actually surprised.

"Yeah, I'm testing the water for you," I said. "I can't remember if I go over or under." I'm sure he couldn't have heard me with the rumble of the jacuzzi jets.

The only reason we can fit in the tub together is that Dave has lost a significant amount of weight. As he climbed into the tub, I was still trying to remember whether my legs went over his or under his. We kind of fit like a pretzel when comfortably situated. I motioned for him to put the tub pillow behind his neck, never missing an opportunity to dote on Dave.

"I wish you could smell how good it smells in here," I told him.

He nodded. Probably because he didn't hear me. Or maybe it was because we're both now used to the fact that for over two years, since having his nose removed, he hasn't been able to smell anything.

Dave leaned his head on the pillow and closed his eyes. I stared at him. The rumble of the jets put me in an almost trance-like state. I continued to stare. I memorized his face—his ears that protrude from the sides of his head more than average, the scars and disfigurement that have been torturing him for the last two years, every detail—knowing I'm not going to be able to feel him this close forever.

He turned the jets off, which were starting to sound obnoxious. It was so quiet. He probably knew I'd start talking; I always talk during these quiet moments. I told him when I tub alone I put my head at the other end, but when I tub with him I sit this way. He asked me why.

"Well, so you don't have the overflow drain in your back," I said. "Plus, now I visualize you at that end. So in the future, when you're not here, I'll sit this way when I want to see your face."

He knows I'm struggling with the idea of him not being here and am grasping at every coping mechanism I can.

I asked him if the days were more important to him now that they're limited.

"I don't think about it," he said. "I think about laying my head on your lap, getting a 'wub' and enjoying the closeness."

We have reached a heightened level of intimacy that few people ever experience in their lifetime. It's something more than love. I don't know if there's a word for it. I really don't know what it is, but I know what it feels like, and I know we never would have gotten here if we didn't know our time was so limited.

*　*　*

It was four years ago, the year before the pandemic. A good friend had urged Dave to run for town council. Dave is one of the most likable people anyone could ever have the privilege of meeting. He's funny, sincere, ethical, and insanely intelligent, and he can talk to people from all realms of life. Everyone walks away from Dave feeling like they're smart, funny, and likable. Who wouldn't like a guy that makes you feel like that?

Anyway, our friends had given Dave the nudge to run for town council. Being that he finds retirement not as enjoyable as I do, he accepted the challenge.

Dave had been having an on-again, off-again frog in his throat. Knowing he'd be doing a fair amount of public speaking, we were concerned that his constant attempt to clear his throat would become a distraction. We scheduled a visit to an ear, nose, and throat doctor to resolve this issue. I don't believe I went to that appointment with Dave. That was before I became "The Mouthpiece." But he told me that Dr. Lichtenstein had run a scope up his nose and down his throat. There was no solid diagnosis, just an observation of mild irritation of the vocal cords. Dave was prescribed various medications over the next few months. Possibly reflux? Possibly sinus drainage? A constantly clogged nose and a throat that never cleared continued to plague him.

Eventually, Dave developed a recurring bloody nostril. This was certainly unusual, but he dealt with this frequent bloody nose by stuffing the one side with tissues and going about his day. Months passed before Dave visited his regular doctor for a routine check-up.

"I'm coming with you, and we're going to get to the bottom of this bloody nose," I say.

We describe the frequency of the nosebleeds to the physician. He suspects Dave has a sore or a cut that's attempting to heal and suggests cauterization will resolve the problem. He does this without any numbing agent. Poor Dave! As the doctor burns the inside of his nose, the lower half of Dave's body lifts off the table as he clenches his butt in pain and scrunches his face.

That was the last time either of us ever saw that physician.

Within weeks, Dave's nostril had started bleeding again, and we concurred that a return visit to the specialist was in order. This was about six or seven months after our initial visit. The prescriptions were having no effect, and Dave's froggy throat wasn't clearing up. We ran through the list of symptoms with Dr. Lichtenstein: Dave's nose was still stuffy, he still had a rasp in his throat that he couldn't clear, and by that time he'd been having this chronic bloody nose for months.

I don't know why I wasn't more persistent that she needed to run some tests. Normally I'm skeptical about everything. But she was a specialist with over thirty years of experience, so I had put my trust in her. **This was my first mistake**.

Dr. Lichtenstein advised us that Dave had a deviated septum, something I dealt with for the first thirty-five years of my life. I had surgery to repair it during the early part of our marriage. Being that it was a game-changer for me, I urged Dave to do the surgery.

Dave had been dealing with chronic nosebleeds for about eight months by the time we finally scheduled the surgery. It was the day after his sixty-seventh birthday. It was also during the height of the pandemic, so family wasn't allowed to stay, even in the waiting room. I had to sit in my car. I remember not being very nervous; Dave was in relatively good health, and this was a routine surgery. When Dave was done, they called me on the phone and said he was moving to recovery. The next call directed me to drive around the side of the building and pick him up.

Since I'd had this surgery twenty years ago, I'd watched several YouTube videos about the improvements made to the nasal packing. I assured Dave that the worst would be the next few days until the packing came out. Then he'd be able to breathe freely. Then everything would be perfect!

I will never forget what happened two days following the surgery.

I've been out of the house, ironically getting my annual mammogram to maintain the health of "my girls." When I return home, Dave tells me the specialist called. She had taken a biopsy of a very normal-looking papilloma during the surgery and the pathology report just came back. It says the biopsy tested positive . . . Dave has cancer.

"What? You have cancer?" I look at him as though he said it's been scientifically proven that the moon is made of green cheese.

If I'd had a crystal ball at that moment, it would have shown me the next three years of our lives would resemble a tornado, followed by eerie bouts of stillness, followed by another tornado.

Dave then told me Dr. Lichtenstein wanted to perform a surgical procedure right away. I called the doctor's office immediately. As soon as I gave my name, I was told Dr. Lichtenstein was expecting my call. Apparently I'd already earned the reputation of The Mouthpiece . . . the patient advocate.

Oddly, I don't remember much of the conversation I had with her. I do remember her pushing to do the surgery on Monday . . . to cut it all out . . . that she'd be taking lots of biopsies and fastidiously labeling them to go to a university hospital about three hours away from us . . . that she recommended we follow up with them. And I do remember Dr. Lichtenstein telling me that although she has biopsied many papillomas, this was the first cancer she's actually encountered.

Why in God's name did I let her go back in his nose? I don't know whether it would have changed the outcome, but she had no business doing cancer surgery. She has three decades of experience yet tells me this is the first cancer she's encountered?!

This was my second mistake, and it would be my last.

Dave had the surgery with her that Monday. The doctor was pleased with herself, saying she'd taken dozens of tissue samples and submitted them to the university hospital. We were able to get appointments scheduled for imaging tests about three weeks later.

When we see the head honcho in the Department of Otolaryngology, he tells us they reviewed all the biopsies and notes from our local specialist. He diagnoses Dave with sinonasal cancer, a rare type of sinus cancer. Fortunately, the type of sinonasal cancer he has is squamous cell carcinoma, the most common of the nasal cancers. It's treatable but can be very aggressive. It doesn't grow like most other cancers. Getting rid of this cancer won't be as simple as cutting out a tumor until you have clear margins. This cancer grows like crabgrass. They can cut it out over here and get clear margins, but there could be more of it over there.

We are given three choices: First choice, surgery; that will give Dave a 40–45 percent chance of remaining cancer-free for five years. Second choice, surgery and radiation; that will double those odds and give us an 80–85 percent chance. Third choice, do nothing; he'll be dead in a year.

It appears to be an easy choice. We choose door number two.

The first surgery is put on the calendar for less than a week out.

The next three years were filled with three surgeries, thirty rounds of radiation, dozens of immunotherapy and chemotherapy infusions, and almost daily oral chemotherapy. Dave lost all sense of taste and most of his salivary glands. He lost his nose after ultimately having to get a full rhinectomy. He lost all his sinuses and almost lost his right eye. He lost all enjoyment of food and eventually the desire and ability to eat, so he also lost one hundred pounds.

What didn't he lose? He didn't lose his sense of humor, his charm, his intelligence, his dignity, or his likability factor. He didn't lose his ability to love and be loved. People were amazed by his perseverance!

He's now living with a hole in his face where his nose used to be. When in public, we keep it covered by his "manhole cover," an irregularly shaped piece of gauze disguised with flesh-colored tape. We fashioned it to fit over the hole that oozes blood and mucus daily. The manhole cover has changed shape as the hole in Dave's face has continued to progress. Dave has no vanity; he wears the cover to make *other* people comfortable.

After Dave's rhinectomy, I started learning about every device that could make Dave's life easier. I researched everything I could about this cancer. I was more than satisfied with our two doctors at the university hospital; between them and our nurse navigator Mario, they were always available to me. We joked that I could teach new residents how to use the patient portal. I emailed them constantly. I advocated for Dave constantly.

I send Dave for massage, acupuncture, and hyperbaric oxygen therapy treatments. When I read the ingredients label on the side of a bottle of adult nutrition, I nearly gag; water, glucose syrup, sugar, and vegetable oil. This is no way to get healthy! I wonder how I can keep Dave's body in good health while he fights cancer.

I complain to the hospital that there's no information regarding the metabolic changes of a cancer patient. I consult with dietitians. I am 100 percent responsible for all of his nutrition. I create "magical shakes." They have anywhere between ten and fifteen ingredients, and I change the ingredients every few months as his preference changes or as I learn new information. Optimally, I need to get two thousand calories in him daily. Cancer steals nutrition. When his cancer spikes, he gets more calories.

Ultimately, we realize we will never cure his cancer. Dave will never be in remission. We accept we will have to settle for managing cancer. We will manage it the best we can.

A month or so ago, we realized we're losing the battle. We realized cancer will take his life. I am certain Dave started accepting his death over a year ago. He's certainly accepting this better than me. Actually, it's quite likely I'm not accepting it at all.

Tuesday, October 3

I was thinking the other day that Dave could use a haircut. I've always loved his hair cut short, nice and clean around the ears and the back of the neck. I'm sure that's how he wore his hair when he was in the air force. Much like the way he still tucks his undershirt into his underwear, it's a military thing that has stuck with him for a lifetime. My dad tucked his undershirt into his underwear till the day he died, albeit a premature death at the age of forty-five.

I know I can trim Dave's hair; I often use the clippers that I use on Sadie to clean up the back of his neck. But I thought it might be nice for him to have a real haircut. He's been so brave about going out in public with his manhole cover on the middle of his face for the last couple of years. It really doesn't faze him. And I'm surprised how many people don't look at his face when walking by. I know this because I watch everyone we walk past. I've grown so protective of Dave. If someone stares at him too long, I change my position to block their view. If I see them look and tell their friend to look, I stare them down. Dave couldn't care less. Actually, when it's children that look at him, he encourages them.

About seven weeks ago, we were on our most recent RV trip and in an adorable town called St. Ignace, Michigan, just a ferry ride away from the infamous Mackinac Island. We set up camp and someone recommended a pizza place for dinner.

Food has been a sketchy subject since Dave's cancer, but he does try to eat when he can, if only to allow me the enjoyment of dining out... another thing lost to cancer.

We're sitting in this pizza place next to the window and there's a deck outside. Very few people are on the deck, as the wind is kicking up and the temps are dropping. There's one family enjoying their meal outside. The adults are sitting back in their seats, have full bellies, and are chatting away. Two children, maybe five and six years old, are running around the deck. The little girl wanders over to the window and presses her face against it, cupping her hands so she can see better. The first thing she sees is Dave. Her eyes widen.

"I think you have a visitor," I say.

Dave looks at the little girl. His eyes widen . . . then he sticks his tongue out.

I sit there shaking my head, thinking, "Why do you encourage this?"

She runs off and a moment later comes back with the little boy, both of them now giggling with their faces scrunched up against the glass. Dave sticks his tongue out again.

I don't know who annoys me more at the moment: the parents for not keeping an eye on their kids, the kids for inserting themselves during our dinner, or my husband for encouraging these shenanigans.

It's silly for me to be annoyed. It's just small shit in the scope of things, and I'm too overprotective.

It wasn't until very recently that Dave's gait changed and he started being uncomfortable out in public. I've told him he clippety-clops along. His right leg is doing something weird. From my perspective, it looks like he's trying to step over a log. I bet it's the fentanyl patch and the liquid morphine combo that's creating this new disability, but I really don't know.

About two weeks ago, I mentioned to Dave that I got an email from CARFAX with an offer to buy his car. I've always found it annoying when I get one of those emails. It'll say, "It's time for an oil change...did you have your tires rotated?" One thing that really pisses me off is when people get in my business. And by "people" I mean anyone.

Dave and I talked about what I should do with his car after he's gone. You know...after he dies. We don't have to use that word all the time, do we? It's not like I'm not aware of where this is leading. But let's just refer to it as "after he's gone" or "when he leaves." Let's make it sound like it's not the most permanent state of being, or not being, in this case.

When I mentioned the email to Dave, he thought we should do it. I called up a local CarMax to make an appointment for me to bring the car in. This was the only property we owned that was solely in Dave's name, and I was wondering whether I'd have any issues. I'd heard that unless you have power of attorney for a title owner, the title owner needs to be there in person. I've been signing this man's name for over twenty years, and it always infuriates me when I'm reminded that technically I'm not supposed to do that. Whatever.

Dave hasn't been out of the house in a week, and I think this little trip to sell the car will be too demanding on him. I tell him not to worry about it. I believe that a death certificate will trump the stupid power of attorney. I can deal with this later...after.

Nope. He's insistent. Let's take care of this now. He wants to do as much as we can now to alleviate my burden later.

I have to agree that thinking "We're selling Dave's car" is so much easier than thinking, "My husband died and now I want to get rid of his car."

I reach out to Nora. Many people have said, "Let me know if there's anything I can do . . . call anytime . . . tell me what you need." Nora means it, and I know that.

I text, "Nora, Dave and I are going to sell his car at Car-Max, can you give us a ride home?"

"Yes. When?" she replies. No hesitation. A good friend.

Dave and I drive to CarMax. The transaction takes about an hour. They test drive and examine the car, offer a price, I accept, Dave signs some papers. Done.

I see Nora pull up in her car. She waits outside.

Before we leave, Dave needs to use the restroom. He clippety-clops along. It's a huge room, and there's only one other customer. There are three times more salespeople than they need today. I watch Dave . . . protectively. When he returns, he sits beside me.

"When I walked across the room I felt like an invalid," he says.

I cringe. I want to cry. I want to protect him. I wish I had walked across the room with him so I could have blocked their view or stared them down. It's quite possible no one noticed anything unusual and they just thought some old guy was walking across the room. But my heart aches for him.

Anyway, knowing Dave needed a haircut, I reached out to two of my closest friends and asked, "Do we know anyone who does hair that can come to the house?"

By the next day, I had a barber's contact info and made arrangements for him to cut Dave's hair at the house. What a nice man! He's done this sort of thing before, coming to a residence when someone was too sick to leave. He said to me on the phone, "This isn't my first rodeo, honey." I chuckled.

He chats with Dave as we stand in the front room of our house, which has our kitchen, dining area, and living room. Two men of a generation before cell phones, the internet, and gaming, from the days when men went to barber shops and chatted with other men about sports, business, gossip, and women. Back in the day, women didn't go into barber shops. They were kind of a man cave before man caves were invented. So, these two gab like girls.

The barber lays out all his tools on the dining room table. Dave sits on a chair over a towel to catch some of the fallen hair.

"How do you like it?" he asks Dave.

"Short!" I say.

Dave smiles. Short it is. Happy wife, happy life.

The barber buzzes and clips and chats. He's very careful around Dave's face. He never stares. I wonder what he's thinking about Dave's manhole cover. He's very gentle and often asks if he's being too rough. Dave tells him he's not. But I know Dave is in pain. I know Dave's face hurts so much that he's started shaving only every other day because just running the razor across his face makes his cheek hurt. I watch the barber gently flick the fluffy brush across Dave's skin to brush away the teeny, clipped hairs. I crinkle my eyes to see if Dave winces. He doesn't.

I know the pain is going to get worse. We've been continuing to increase the dosage of the fentanyl patches. I wonder whether Dave will make a conscious decision when he's ready to go, a decision that he's just done, and then he will stop eating and drinking and will require heavy meds. Meds so heavy that he will slip into unconsciousness right before my eyes, so heavy that I wonder if he can hear my words. Or will it be gradual? Will it be like now? Just little by little being more drugged . . . eventually not getting out of bed . . . taking in less nutrition and fewer fluids . . . sleeping more. Will it just be so gradual that one day his heart . . . just . . . stops? Have we said everything that needs to be said? I know we have. I have visualized this moment more times than I can count.

The haircut looked terrific and Dave was pleased. Of course, Dave has always been easy to please. My mind questioned whether Dave would ever get another haircut before . . . he goes. I got a quick flash in my mind's eye of a mortician snipping little hairs from around Dave's ears.

When I thanked the barber and asked how much we owed him, he wouldn't accept any money. He said he does these visits to make things a little easier and to please call again if we need his services. He packed up his bags and was gone.

After he left, I headed to the gym. It was my second time this week. I insisted Dave show me he had his phone on his person. "Call me if *anything* happens," I demanded.

He promised he would.

I decided to hit the heavy bag today, so I tossed my boxing gloves and wraps into my gym bag. I've never boxed before, but I enjoy shadowboxing. There have been so many times I've felt anger well up inside of me over the last three years. I often think I'd like to take a baseball bat to the pilings that hold my beach house fourteen feet above sea level. Being that I overthink everything, I've considered that actually doing this would really hurt my body and I'd look like a lunatic. Besides,

I don't own a baseball bat. I'll never actually do it, but just thinking about how good it would feel to whack the crap out of something is somehow stress-relieving.

I warmed up on the treadmill, then wrapped my hands. I stood in front of the heavy bag and imagined cancer, a big C painted on the front of the bag. Jab . . . jab . . . cross . . . hook . . . dance . . . jab . . . cross . . . hook . . . hook . . . hook. Anyone looking at me must have wondered what this poor bag did to me. My heart rate monitor told me I was working too hard. *Huffing . . . puffing . . . shit . . . why can't I keep going . . . I have to breathe . . . I'm out of breath.* I beat on the bag for four rounds of two minutes, with a short rest between rounds. I thought of real boxers and how many rounds they're able to keep moving. What amazing conditioning!

Just as I was taking the gloves off, I felt a tap on my right shoulder. I turned and saw it was Karina! Karina runs the gym and has been my trainer over the years. She's also my friend. We've shared many personal stories about husbands, mothers, life . . . we've shared it all. I haven't seen her in a while, though, not since Dave started hospice and I stopped going to the gym regularly. I didn't see her earlier this week when I went, but I'd had a mutual friend call her to let her know Dave wasn't doing well. I just didn't have the energy to go through the story once again.

Karina is Catholic and has strong faith. I envy that. Maybe faith is something you have to work at, like conditioning for a boxing match. Maybe it doesn't just happen. Maybe you have to make it happen.

We talked about how I'm doing and how Dave is doing. She's one of the only people I know who might actually share "that thing" with her husband like Dave and I do—that thing that is greater than love. I told her that. I told her there's something more than love between Dave and me, a feeling that has no word to describe it. I also told her she has that with her husband. The second she said she couldn't imagine life without him, she started to cry. Just the thought is painful for her.

Karina and I talked about two other people from the gym, people she cares a great deal about, and the awful things going on in their lives. One is a young mother whose child recently died in an accident, and the other is a young man whose brain cancer has metastasized. Fucking cancer.

She told me she questions God why this is all happening. Why are good people suffering and dying? What's the plan? She has faith in God that it will be okay, that everything happens for a reason. I am not so confident.

I questioned her, "What if this is all there is?"

"NO!" she boomed. "It's not!" She is sure there is more. She is sure we will be reunited with those we love. I hope she's right.

Sometime after I returned from the gym, Myra came for her second visit of the week. I've grown to like Myra, the Scorpio. She jokes about us both being Scorpios. Maybe that's why she has a read on me. Maybe it's because she's been doing this job long enough to know the mindset of a caregiver. Maybe she just cares about people.

I think of how upset I was when I found out Myra would be taking personal time in October. I've come to learn that she has thyroid cancer and needs to have her thyroid removed. This Thursday is her surgery. She's as bubbly and light-hearted as ever, and it's the usual routine: vitals, pain level, anything new?

Myra told me she's proud of me for going to the gym. And not for the normal reasons you'd be supportive of someone going to the gym but because I'd left Dave for a couple of hours and taken care of myself. She knows I don't want to leave his side. But she also knows I need to take care of my mind and body during this time because caregiver burnout is a real thing.

We chatted about exercise, her experience with Weight Watchers, and general health stuff. Jessica will be her replacement while she recovers from her surgery. I'm looking forward to Myra's return . . . my fellow Scorpio. It's amusing that my tune has changed about her returning after her surgery. I don't normally change my mind that easily. I guess she has successfully wooed me.

Dave and I certainly spend more time talking about important stuff these days, but we try to maintain some normalcy with routine chitchat. I think I've become a better listener lately. With me normally speaking 90 percent of the time and Dave speaking the remainder, it would stand to reason that I don't have a whole lot of experience listening. Generally, when Dave speaks it's not just words; it's real thoughts. He never babbles.

Tonight, after watching TV and while snuggling for a bit on the couch, he complimented me on something. Then the conversation drifted to another subject. Always loving a good compliment, I said with a smirk on my face, "Now, can you tell me more about what I'm good at?" I didn't really need to hear a compliment, but I always value one that comes from Dave.

He said, "You do everything good. I don't know how anybody does this without somebody like you, and yet I don't think anyone has someone like you."

I gently kissed his cheek and rested my head on his shoulder. I said nothing.

Saturday, October 7

*T*onight I took Sadie for her usual after-dinner beach walk. It's late in the season, so there were very few people on the beach. I allowed Sadie off her leash only because I've trained her well.

Shortly into our walk, I saw her heading over to a woman sitting on a staircase that crosses the dune. I don't normally allow my dogs to approach strangers; you never know who might be afraid or have allergies. As Sadie approached her, I walked over to ask if she was okay with the visit. We started to make polite conversation, and within thirty seconds she mentioned her husband recently passed. Hmm. She didn't get choked up, but I could still see the hurt in her eyes.

I told her my husband is at home and that hospice is coming to our house. I teared up a bit and my voice became croaky.

She had that look on her face, the one that told me she knew what my future will become. She said, "Cancer?"

I nodded.

She patted the step next to her, offering me a seat. I took it. We sat for an hour and a half. She told me about her life with Jim and how abruptly it had ended, one month ago yesterday . . . the day before my twenty-first wedding anniversary. Yesterday was her wedding anniversary. She's here because she wanted to go someplace she had never been with Jim so that there wouldn't be any memory triggers. I knew that was impossible, but I also knew what she meant.

I told her all about Dave. I told her how he's my hero...how I've fiercely advocated for him for three years...how he's the only person in this world who has truly taken care of me...how I'm so afraid of life without him...how I don't have any strong belief of what happens next. Heaven? Nothing? Something in between?

We took turns talking. Our stories are so similar, yet so different. When I told her my stories, she laughed, not just because they were funny but because of the ironic similarities to hers. She's one year younger than I am, she's talkative, and she's been a caregiver and advocate for someone she loves. She's a widow. She seemed strong...something everyone tells me I am.

I told her about the butterfly dress. I told her a little about Gingey Bean. I told her Dave told me to buy a "comfy Hawaiian jumper" for his funeral so I went online looking for a dress. She said she hadn't been able to bear to go to the store to shop for dresses either, so she'd selected among three she'd bought online. I knew exactly what she meant. I showed her a picture of the off-white dress with the red, blue, and black butterflies that I'll wear. She said, "It'll look great with your coloring."

During moments of silence, I remembered a one-sided conversation I'd had in my car a couple of weeks ago.

I just walked out of the pharmacy. I'm here again to pick up more hospice medications. It's one of the many times of the day when I appear to be handling business as usual, but there's turmoil going on inside. I get in my car and start crying. I look through the windshield and up at the sky, calling out to my dad who I lost when I was a child, then to my friend Lisa who died way too young.

"If you love me...if you ever loved me...if there's anyone up there who loves me...please give me a sign. Give

me a sign that it will be okay, that there's something after this and I don't need to be scared."

I feel some immediate relief, partially from the heavy cry and partially because I feel like I don't need to "do" any-thing now. I did my part. I asked. Now I wait.

A couple of days pass, and I tell Dave the story of me in the car shouting up towards the sky. I'm frustrated and sad because there's been no sign.

In his infinite wisdom, Dave says, "There's still time."

I silently started to wonder whether this lady sitting next to me was my sign. I told her about my request for a sign and my crying jag in the pharmacy parking lot. She knew exactly what I was talking about—going from zero to ten on the crying scale within thirty seconds. Just as I started to tell her I thought she might be my sign, she said she was wondering whether she's my sign. We both paused and stared at the ocean. Hmm. For real? Could her being at this place and at this time be more than a coincidence?

"I don't know why I called your dog over," she said.

"You called Sadie over? I didn't hear that."

"Yeah, I saw you and your dog. I thought she was a cute dog, and you looked deep in thought. I hope it wasn't a bad thing calling her over." She has a rescue named Sophie, so she likes dogs.

After a while, it started getting dark and chilly. She asked if I wanted to exchange numbers. I told her I felt like we should. Even if we never talk again, I'm afraid three months from now I'll want to reach out to "that lady on the beach" and never know how to get in touch with her. I sent her a text telling her my name. She replied with her name: Chris.

I walked her back to the house she was staying at for the weekend. Oddly enough, it's the other half of a duplex where

Dave and I have friends. We hugged, both of us still puzzled that she may be my sign.

When I left Chris, I was only about five minutes from home. I walked briskly with Sadie; it was cold and I was excited to tell Dave I may have gotten my sign. That made me think about how I'm going to have so many times in my future when I will want to rush home and talk to Dave but he will no longer be there.

I texted Chris during the short walk home and told her I was excited to tell Dave she may be my sign. She suggested telling him may make him feel better too, knowing that the universe gave me a sign and that I'm going to be okay . . . especially knowing that I'll be okay.

I burst into the doorway, and Dave asked where I'd been. He'd been looking at the Find My app on his phone, wondering why I hadn't moved for an hour and a half. I told him all about Chris and Jim. While we were talking, I felt my phone vibrate with a text. I ignored it and continued talking to Dave. I thought I saw a smidgen of peace on his face as I considered Chris-from-the-beach might be a sign.

I headed off to shower before we sat down to our nightly ritual of an evening snack and a bit of television. I looked at the waiting text and saw it was from Chris. She had mentioned a book she was reading, one that was giving her some comfort, helping her believe there is something after this life. She sent me a screenshot of the book cover and said to look at the upper-right corner. There in the corner was a beautiful blue butterfly. If I hadn't told her about the dress I'll be wearing for Dave's funeral, she wouldn't have given the butterfly a second thought.

I rushed into that back bedroom we call an office. It's a feel-good room where I've been keeping many tchotchkes that make me smile, things that have been given to me over the years, mostly by Dave. I walked to the wall on the left and took a picture of an object Dave bought me fifteen years ago. It's a block of Lucite, and inside of it is a beautiful blue butterfly.

Sunday, October 8

I woke up at 4:45 this morning after having a nightmare. I've always been a vivid dreamer and have woken up to many nightmares since childhood. For as long as I've been married to Dave, I've often "accidentally" woken him up shortly after waking from my nightmare. "I had a nightmare," I'll say. "What was it about?" he'll ask while wrapping an arm around me. Often, through tears, I'll tell him all the details of the dream. I think he's never understood why I cry once I'm awake and know the dream wasn't real. The poor guy often fights to stay awake while I recall the upsetting details, then offers his words of comfort.

Today was a little different. I woke and thought about the wildness of the dream. Being pretty good at interpreting my dreams, I started to pick it apart. I did not "accidentally" wake Dave today. He needed to sleep. It's the only time he feels no pain.

As I lay there thinking about the dream, I realized the temperature had dropped during the night and the room was cold. I got up to close the window. We have windows on either side of the bed, and usually it's just mine that's open. It squeaked as I lowered it. I slipped back under the covers, and Dave started to stir. He got up and went to the bathroom.

When he came back, I said, "I had a nightmare."

As he took the position of the "big spoon" enveloping my body, he asked what it was about. I told him all the details I could remember. With the very last sentence, I started to cry.

He squeezed me tighter. "That's my Snookums ... my very best Snookums ... she's the best Snookums in the world," he quietly sang.

Dave quickly fell back to sleep while I tossed and turned for a couple more hours. I finally got out of bed just after sunrise. After my first cup of coffee, I took Sadie for a walk. I was thinking about my conversation with Chris-from-the-beach and all the similarities of our lives, as well as the blue butterfly.

I remembered Chris telling me how she doesn't like looking at Jim's empty pillow, so she stuffs his hat with socks and sets it atop his pillow. When we were speaking, she pulled out her phone to show me a picture of him with the hat on. He was wearing a bucket hat.

"He wore a bucket hat?" I asked. "Dave wore a bucket hat."

I hated that bucket hat. Dave wore it when we went to Hawaii . . . so many years ago. Since then, he's been wearing a newer, somewhat adorable, bucket hat with the name of our friend's coffee shop on it. Then I remembered the baseball cap Chris was holding the whole time we sat on the stairs.

When Dave and I first met, I was a sheriff's officer working in the legal division. I served and executed all types of court papers, including summonses, writs, and restraining orders. Dave was the president of a small, local oil company. Eventually he started working at a larger one, retiring as Chief Operating Officer.

I'd been routinely serving papers on Dave's company. They hadn't done anything wrong, but they'd been holding judgments on property that was in foreclosure. When I first met Dave, I was thirty years old and he was forty-one. For years I asked to see Dave at the front desk, hoping he'd be there because he was so professional with receiving the papers. So many people gave me a lot of flak at the time of service. For years I passed through his office quickly, in and out in only a moment, without any personal conversation.

Probably about five or six years into my popping in and out of his office, we started chatting. He told me he had three children, two boys in their early twenties and a daughter who was getting ready to leave for college. I had no interest in dating Dave, but I did think he was funny and enjoyed our conversations when I was in his office. And he was so personable! The way he could make me feel like I was the only person in the room was magic. I didn't realize at the time that he exerts that magic on everyone he speaks to.

Email was just getting popular at the time, and "You've got mail" was becoming a household phrase. When I told Dave I bought my first personal computer, he suggested exchanging email addresses. We wrote back and forth, me usually talking about my house or my dogs. I knew that Dave was engaging in person, but I came to realize that he's downright magnetic with the written word! His emails were masterpieces that left me chuckling and eagerly replying so I'd get another email. I remember really looking forward to them.

Dave was very successful at his job. He often qualified to win a one-week trip sponsored by a large petroleum corporation, and it was always to some five-star resort at a magnificent location. On top of that, he annually attended another trip that was usually four days long, always at a Ritz-Carlton, and typically involved only one meeting; the rest of the time was for pleasure.

During the coldest part of winter 2001, Dave mentioned to me he was competing for a week-long trip to Hawaii. His daughter had left for college the previous fall and he didn't have a lady friend at the time, so if he won this trip he wouldn't have a traveling companion.

Hmmm. He's such a nice guy and so funny ... maybe he'll wanna take me.

For the next month, I nonchalantly interjected in my emails to Dave how I hate New Jersey winters and would just love to be someplace warm, if only for a few days. After weeks of this, Dave sent me a very cautiously worded email explaining he has an upcoming trip: He didn't want to scare me off, we could go as friends, it would be fun, the trip is for four days . . . in Jamaica.

Jamaica?! What the hell happened to Hawaii? Anyone can go to Jamaica!

I agreed to go. About a week or so later, I got another very carefully worded email from Dave. He had been nurturing our business-turning-personal relationship for seven years and didn't want to blow it by scaring me off.

> *"I'm going to ask you a question," he says. "No matter what the answer is, please don't cancel Jamaica."*
>
> *He tells me he won the trip to Hawaii and asks if I'd like to go. It's on the island of Lanai, top-notch all the way. The trip costs an absolute fortune and we won't have to pay a dime.*
>
> *Thinking of the adage about actions speaking louder than words, I should say no to his offer. Is this guy going to believe I have no romantic interest in him if I agree to be his companion for two trips?*
>
> *The plan is to go to Hawaii for a week, come home for about ten days, then head off to Jamaica for four days.*
>
> *"I'll do it!"*

Dave was a complete gentleman in Hawaii, and the trip was exceptional. The entire week was filled with moments we will remember and relive for a lifetime. We had adventures we never could have afforded to have on our own, ate food I didn't even know could taste so good, and laughed harder than I thought possible. It was the kind of laughter where you're doubled over, holding your stomach in pain, shouting, "Stop making me laugh!"

But one of my favorite moments occurred very quietly and happened almost daily.

Dave has never been a beach person. With his Irish complexion, he can get a sunburn from a full moon. When we didn't have an excursion planned in the afternoons, I'd head to the beach for a couple of hours while Dave hung out in the room and read his book.

When I'd return from the beach, I'd always have lots to say. I wanted to tell him about everything and everyone I saw in his absence. I'd flop across the bed on my stomach to face his chair. He always put his book down. He always made me feel like whatever little stories I wanted to share were the most important things he heard each day, just like he did when I chatted with him in his office.

After a week we returned home. I thought about how genuinely nice and kind Dave was, but I still didn't see us as a couple. Ten days passed and we were ready to leave for Jamaica. Dave made sure there was no chance his snoring would keep me awake on this trip. Unbeknownst to me, he had upgraded us to a suite at the Ritz-Carlton so I'd have my own bedroom. He personally paid big bucks for that upgrade for sure, but he implied that the company had taken care of it.

The first day was a travel day and uneventful. The second day we spent some time going downtown. Being the chairman of some kind of board, Dave had to speak to a roomful of people that afternoon. He told me I couldn't come because I'd make him nervous if I were in the room. *I would? But not the roomful of people?* So I went to the beach, lay by the pool, and visited the gift shop, where I charged an adorable Ritz-Carlton sweatsuit to the room. The third day? The third day was the magical day. The third day was the day that changed both our lives forever.

We plan an excursion to ride down a gentle river on a guided bamboo raft. I'm still cautious to not sit too close to Dave. I'm pretty sure he likes me, and I'm afraid of giving him the wrong signal. When the guide offers to take our picture, we sit close and Dave puts his arm around me. As soon as the picture is taken, I wiggle a couple of inches back to where I was sitting.

At the end of the guided tour is a rum-tasting party. I like rum! We drink shots of quality rum . . . several shots. I guess that's exactly what I need . . . something to help me let my guard down a bit, something to relax those walls I've solidly reinforced for so many years. With a few hours left before we need to dress for dinner, we take a shuttle back to our suite.

This fantastic, fancy suite is on a corner of the building with gorgeous ocean views on two sides. The bedroom, where I sleep, and the living room, where Dave sleeps, both have balconies. Oddly enough, this perfectly appointed room with two balconies that costs a fortune has only one lounge chair on only one of the balconies.

Feeling rather happy after the rum-tasting event, I grab the bottle of Mad Annie's rum that's in our room and bring it out to the balcony to where Dave is sitting. I sit on the chair with him, Dave sitting back in the lounger with me sitting in front of him leaning against his chest. We drink delicious creamy rum and talk about our lives for hours. Dave gently scratches my back and my walls come down. My internal walls. After seven years of knowing me, he starts to earn my trust, something I haven't completely given to anyone in a very, very long time.

After hours of enjoying this close conversation, we shower separately and dress for dinner. I choose to wear a long, black sundress with huge, hot-pink flowers. I'm excited knowing that tonight will be the night the platonic friendship is left in the dust. I wonder whether Dave is feeling the same. The dinner is wonderful as the anticipation builds, and the rest of the night is all it was intended to be.

The next morning is our fourth and last day, a travel day. We sit closely at the airport, nuzzling and holding hands. When we see other couples from the trip, I wonder whether they can tell. Do they know we were friends at the start of this trip and now we're so much more?

After our flight, Dave drives me home. I walk inside and call my mother to let her know I've safely arrived home. I also tell her, "Mom, I think this is the guy I'm gonna marry."

Ironically, Dave thinks our evening of romance will probably be a one-time event, likely encouraged by the amount of rum we enjoyed.

Still walking on the beach with Sadie, I looked at the staircase I sat on with Chris last night. I thought of the ball cap she was holding, the one her husband wore when he wasn't wearing his bucket hat, the one that had the name of his favorite place embroidered on the front of it. The hat that read, "Jamaica."

10

Thursday, October 12

*M*egan has been here visiting since the beginning of the week and is driving home to Florida today. She's married now and has three high-maintenance children, along with a demanding job as an attorney. Being his daughter, she's also the apple of Dave's eye.

Last month, she made the drive up here three times, bringing each of her children for a weekend so they could spend special time with their grandpa. Dave hates the wear and tear she puts on herself by driving over nine hours week after week, but he realizes she's a grown woman and is doing what she needs to do.

Dave and Megan have always been extremely close. James and his brother Patrick were out of the house by the time Megan went into high school, so she had a lot of one-on-one time with her dad. I remember Dave often talking about Megan whenever I'd stop in his office to serve him papers. She's naturally athletic and played quite a bit of traveling soccer in high school. Dave was a true "soccer dad" and often shared with me the time and location of an upcoming weekend soccer match. I never went to any of them, and Megan was a freshman in college by the time we met. She was home on break when Dave and I needed that ride to the airport for our trip to Hawaii.

It was less than a month later that Dave and I were seriously involved. We spent weekends visiting Megan at college, but from early on it was obvious there was some conflict between us. I imagine that's to be expected when a love interest enters the picture of a daddy–daughter relationship as close as theirs. Megan and I were the only ones who felt any conflict; Dave was happily oblivious to it for many, many years.

My relationship with Megan became closer after she graduated from college and got married. She's eighteen years my junior, so technically she could be my daughter, but I wouldn't say we have a mother–daughter relationship. In both of our experiences, that's probably a good thing. Megan and I have had unhealthy relationships with our mothers, so a mother–daughter relationship is not exactly something for us to strive for. I imagine we're somewhere between close sisters and extremely close friends.

Dave has excelled at being a caring, supportive father, often jumping into the car to rush to his kids during times of trouble. Megan has certainly picked up that trait from her father, often making the long drive during this cancer nightmare. She's been present during most of Dave's surgeries, and each time she attempted to care for me, the caregiver, while I impatiently waited for progress reports from Dr. Thorn.

This last trip of Megan's was solo—no kids. We've spent a lot of time together since Dave sleeps a lot, but during the week I've tried to give them ample time alone, believing this will be the last time they see each other.

Megan and I have definitely ruffled each other's feathers over these last three years. We're both smart, strong women and love Dave fiercely, and sometimes that creates conflict. Unfortunately, poor Dave has been in the middle, but he's done an outstanding job in his attempts to validate our feelings without degrading the other's position. He's able to do this because he loves us both so deeply and doesn't want either of us to be hurt. He also knows there will come a time when Megan and I will have only each other to lean on.

Halfway into her visit, Megan and I were working out on the back deck, "getting our fitness on," as she calls it. "You and I handle this so differently," she said. "You want to get rid of everything that reminds you of him, and I want to keep everything."

I don't think she knew how her words stung. I explained that we're taking care of the practical tasks. "Dad said it would be easier for me to adjust to his car being sold while he's still living than after he dies," I told her.

"But I would've bought his car from you," she replied, "just because it belonged to him."

Although it appears to her I've been cleaning out her father's things, I'm really just organizing. She would probably be shocked to know that upon Dave's death, I likely won't be able to move or remove anything.

She told me they were driving somewhere, just the two of them, when they both acknowledged they didn't need to have some big father–daughter end-of-life talk; they've said all the words they need to say. I was happy to hear this, and it doesn't surprise me knowing the relationship they've had.

Dave has already told Megan that at the time of his death, he would rather she be at an amusement park where they shared great memories with her kids than here at the house. He doesn't want her to remember him like he will be at the end. And at this time, I believe I would prefer to be alone when Dave dies.

Before she drove home, we all went out to a great restaurant where they serve terrific Thai and Vietnamese food. Dave even commented that because there were many customers of Asian descent dining there, the food must be close to authentic. The three of us hadn't been out in a restaurant in a very long time, and it stirred up memories of happier days.

Dave ate surprisingly well, and Megan and I rode the high of his appearing to feel better than usual. Dave picked up the tab on "his" credit card, something he often does when his kids visit or when he takes me out for a special birthday or anniversary dinner.

Just before we headed to the car to go home, Megan took pictures of me and Dave on the restaurant's brightly decorated porch. I didn't know it at the time, but these would be the last pictures of me and Dave together.

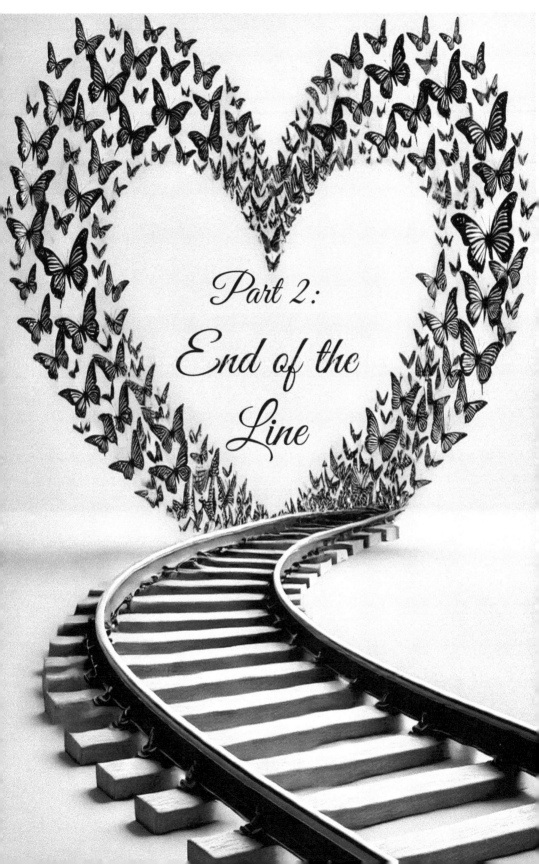

Part 2:

End of the

Line

Sunday, October 15

A roller coaster is a really accurate description of what the last three years have been like. That slow crawl to the top filled with suspense is much like our three-hour drives to the hospital for scans: filled with anticipation and some fear. The rush to the bottom when you're screaming and can barely breathe? That's like the times we've gotten bad news. And the times when the ride is just rolling along at high speeds, dangerously taking curves until the next rise or fall? That's when we were cruising along, beating the crap out of cancer.

Having the ride span three years has allowed a little time to emotionally adjust to each stage. But what about at the end when we have to ride the entire ride in a span of forty-eight hours?

Somehow, I thought that hospice and death were going to be smooth, predictable experiences. I thought they would involve pain management provided by hospice followed by a sleep Dave never wakes from. I know that sounds clinical, but taking the emotion out of the whole subject and just considering the physical events is what I'm good at, and that's what I thought this would be. I thought Dave's medication would increase to the point that sleep took over his days and nights. Then, one morning, he wouldn't wake up. He would quietly exhale and never inhale again. I expected I would wake one morning to find my darling Dave beside me without life. That in itself would be traumatizing and painful. But that does not describe the final two weeks of Dave's life.

Not. At. All.

Since September 18, Dave's pain medication has consisted of fentanyl patches and liquid, concentrated morphine. Both drugs have been routinely adjusted according to Dave's pain level. For each patient in hospice, this is a balancing act. For Dave, he wants to maintain just enough clear-headedness for his visitors. He doesn't want to sleep all day, and he doesn't want to completely sacrifice his quality of life for pain management. We're continuing to tweak the doses of pain meds in a tedious balancing act.

One of the consequences of pain medication is constipation. Although for most of us, an occasional bout of constipation can be easily remedied, for a hospice patient who's eating and drinking very little, this is much more challenging, and the consequences are far more dire. Dave has been taking laxatives when needed. Several days will pass without him having a bowel movement, then eventually he'll have several bouts of diarrhea in one day. I've spoken with one of the triage nurses about how I can better manage this new balancing act of constipation and diarrhea. She explained to me the dangers of constipation in a hospice patient in vivid detail.

The first concern is fecal impaction. This means that Dave's feces could get so packed in his large intestine that it wouldn't be able to move through his body. Having diarrhea wouldn't necessarily mean he'd be free from the worries of a fecal impaction because if the feces were fluid enough to travel around the impaction, we might not know he has one. The hospice nurse would remove a fecal impaction by performing a manual disimpaction, which essentially involves inserting a gloved finger or possibly an enema into Dave's rectum. The next level of concern would be an impaction so severe that Dave could potentially vomit feces. If his constipation reaches that level, he will need to be transported to the hospice center and provided with such a high level of pain management that he will remain unconscious until his natural death.

I was standing on the beach walking Sadie when I had this phone conversation with the triage nurse. I was terrified of these complications on so many levels. I've shared pretty much everything with Dave regarding his health, information I've obtained, and possible complications, but vomiting feces is not one I'm going to mention.

During one of Myra's visits, she brought up the issue of constipation and the possibility of impaction as well as remedies. She didn't go into any detail about vomiting feces, but I saw the look of disgust and concern on Dave's face when she spoke of the manual disimpaction.

"You know, when Elisabeth Kübler-Ross wrote about death with dignity, I don't think this was what she had in mind," Dave said to Myra. He asked how one reconciles a person dying with dignity while a medical person uses a digit to clear a fecal impaction; isn't this a complete violation of someone's dignity?

Myra assured us there are many remedies available before symptoms progress to that point. She also suggested we might benefit, at some point, from a hospital bed.

I could see the anxiety growing on Dave's face, and he's someone who has never appeared anxious to me a day in his life. That couldn't have been obvious to Myra, just to someone who's been married to him for twenty-one years.

"The bed isn't a requirement, right Myra?" I asked her.

She confirmed she was just advising what equipment was available to us and that we'd get only the medical equipment we desire; nothing will be forced on us.

After Myra left, I reminded Dave, "We run this show. You and me. We are a team, and we decide what we want and don't want. If you don't want a hospital bed, no one will be bringing a hospital bed into this house."

He seemed satisfied with my stubborn response.

Dave and I desperately want him to spend his remaining days in our home, so the importance of maintaining regular bowel movements has just moved up considerably. The log-book I've been using to journal Dave's pain medication now includes notes regarding the time and consistency of his bowel movements. When Dave goes to the bathroom, he waits to flush until I can look at it. As humiliating as this may be for Dave, it's a necessary evil.

On a prior occasion, I suggested to Dave that a supposi-tory could be helpful and he wouldn't have to deal with drink-ing any disgusting medicine. He said no. A flat no. But now his constipation has reached a severe concern, so he said we should do it. I'm relieved he brought it up.

What I've come to realize is that Dave's reluctance for the suppository has nothing to do with his modesty and every-thing to do with him not wanting his wife to have to undertake such a task. Dave is more concerned about me being uncom-fortable than himself feeling violated. It's a simple fifteen-second adventure, and afterward I tell him we've reached a new level of intimacy, trying to add some levity. I am well aware that this is the same man who wants the bathroom door closed when he's going number two and doesn't want to talk through the door. I know this is awful for him.

Monday, October 16

Before bed last night, I put Dave's nighttime pills in a pill cup, premeasured the liquid morphine in a syringe, and placed it on Dave's nightstand. At 2 a.m., I helped him take his meds. At 6 a.m., I measured out another dose of meds and walked around to Dave's side of the bed to wake him. I smelled something unusual. I thought it was urine; I figured maybe he'd slept so soundly with these heavy opioids that he'd urinated in his sleep. When I pulled back his covers while he was still slumbering, I could see the discoloration on the sheets.

I gently woke him up. While he lay there looking up at me, I was dreading what I had to tell him but knew I couldn't procrastinate the moment any longer. "I have good news and bad news for you," I said.

He stared at me, waiting to see which news I'd share first.

"The good news is we don't have to worry about you being constipated anymore," I said with a smile. Then I continued: "The bad news is you had a BM during your sleep." It makes me cringe to think how sad this makes him.

The sheets and blankets needed to be washed, although they weren't terribly soiled. The worst part was watching my poor husband head off to the shower with his dirty underwear clinging to his tiny body. He's weak and shaky, and his body is becoming so fragile and thin. It looks like his bones will snap if he bumps himself in the doorway.

As I rushed around grabbing linens to toss in the wash and make a fresh bed, Dave was doing the best he could at cleanup and called me in to help.

"Did I miss anything?" he asked, afraid to twist and turn in a slippery shower.

"Just a tiny spot on the back of your leg," I said, though there was actually a river of brown entangled in his leg hair. I attempted to play down the incident while I rinsed him off, but I knew this was devastating to Dave.

By the time he came out of the bathroom, the bed was made and the dirty laundry was in the washing machine. He walked over to me and said, "I'm sorry."

"Dave," I replied, "you never have to say you're sorry for this. This isn't your fault." I'm heartbroken that he feels he needs to apologize to me.

As far as pain management, I'm feeling like Wonder Woman. This last weekend I played like a scientist, adjusting and logging medication tweaks and ultimately coming up with a combination to substantially reduce Dave's pain by adding ibuprofen. Back when his pain first started, I don't even remember when, probably two years ago, we had a lot of success managing it with ibuprofen.

Jessica came this afternoon and I was excited to tell her about the pain relief. I was not excited to have to tell her that Dave had a nighttime bowel accident.

Tonight while watching television, Dave's hands started jerking, almost like little spasms. I didn't understand why. We assumed it was the opioids. I could see his body tense and release with each tremor. I played a meditation app for us and ran Dave a hot bath. He clippety-clopped down the hall with his new gait, which is worsening. I hoped tucking him in bed all snuggly warm would bring him a good Tuesday.

Tuesday, October 17

Unfortunately, this morning greeted Dave with another bowel movement during the night. He ultimately stayed in bed until 2 p.m., canceling coffee with Colonel Tom, who's been coming to the house for coffee since Dave has been too weak to make the trek to our favorite coffee shop. Tom is leaving for Hawaii on Wednesday, and I really hoped the two could spend some time together.

A few years ago, back when Dave was running for town council, he ran a clean campaign. He used social media platforms to share his positions on topics such as infrastructure and beach management instead of slinging mud at other candidates. Unfortunately, he wasn't able to break through the glass ceiling of Southern, small-town politics. But because of his intelligent campaign and gentle demeanor, Dave got noticed by an alderman of a neighboring beach town who recommended him for a position as Interim Town Manager.

Back when we were living in New Jersey, Dave stepped away from the oil business for about a year and took a position as Town Manager in the town where we lived. So he actually did have some experience with municipal government. Dave interviewed and was offered the job.

A week or so after he started, a different alderman, whose name was Tom, asked Dave about a United States Air Force lapel pin Dave was wearing on his jacket at the time of his interview. The pin caught Tom's eye because his dad was a career air force officer and pilot, and Tom had grown up living on air force bases. Upon talking, the two of them discovered they had common ground with Whiteman Air Force Base in Knob Noster, Michigan. Dave had skipped a grade of school and at age seventeen was particularly young to be graduating from high school and joining the air force; his mother had to sign a permission slip so he could enlist. He was assigned as a combat targeting technician with top-secret clearance. Tom was a high school student at the time and was living on the base because of his dad. It didn't take much conversation for these two to realize they'd dated girls who lived on opposite sides of the same duplex.

Dave and Tom had never actually known each other back in the early '70s when they were both at Whiteman. Dave left Missouri after his enlistment, and Tom ultimately joined the United States Marine Corps, retiring as a colonel in 2008. Fifty years later, they met for the first time, and the history they shared at Whiteman provided the start of a budding bromance.

Meanwhile, after a relatively short time, the mayor and alderman realized they should stop interviewing other Town Manager candidates and offered Dave the permanent position of Town Manager. Dave has always had an amazing ability to create a cohesive, friendly environment wherever he's worked. He spent a little over a year at this job and loved every minute of it before having to resign due to the side effects of his cancer treatment. That's when Tom, who we often affectionately call Colonel Tom, started having coffee dates with Dave on a regular basis.

While sitting at our favorite coffee shop one day, Tom and Dave had daydreamed about visiting Whiteman again and creating their own little bucket-list trip. Tom's wife and I urged the boys to plan and execute this trip sooner rather than later. It was like angels were their escorts, because the trip couldn't have gone any better! The airmen at Whiteman pulled out all the stops for this visiting former airman who has terminal cancer and his retired USMC Colonel buddy.

One doesn't expect to meet a BFF in your late sixties, but when someone comes along with shared values and shared history, sometimes all the dots connect. Dave will forever be known as "Tom's wingman."

I'm starting to feel comfortable getting back to my normal schedule of going to the gym a few days a week and running out for groceries or a trip to the drugstore. But today I didn't feel it would be wise. I'm uncomfortable leaving Dave alone, yet I know he doesn't want me to call a friend over to "old-man-sit." Other than taking a couple of walks with Sadie, moving forward I will not leave the house for anything else.

Eventually, after Dave got out of bed, he plucked away at his computer. I tried to think of this as just a little hurdle, a little low before the next high. He hadn't taken in any nutrition all day, so I managed to find something appealing for him to eat in the evening.

I am completely out of sorts. It's funny how after all these years of marriage I'm still surprised when Dave knows I'm not feeling like my normal self.

He comes by the chair I'm sitting in, the pink one, ruffles my hair, and asks, "What's up with my Snookums?"

"I'm good," I tell him.

He knows better.

Later, while sitting on the couch, I tell him that something he said bothered me. It was nonsense and trivial. So much so that I was angry with myself that I would even get annoyed.

"My poor Snookums," he says. "You see me declining rapidly today and it's tearing you apart. I hate that you have to go through this."

I actually hadn't considered that to be the reason I was triggered, but he hit the nail on the head—as usual. I think it hasn't really clicked in my mind that Dave is declining. I've been so focused on his comfort and treatment that I've never really contemplated that this roller coaster ride is eventually going to end very abruptly.

Dave still had the twitches tonight. We enjoyed a relatively normal night of television and then went to bed. I'll be getting him up at 2 a.m. to help him take his meds again. It seems to be effective at preventing him from waking for the day in tremendous pain.

Wednesday, October 18

I barely slept, waking at midnight, then at 1 a.m., then just giving up on sleep and lying awake. At 1:45, I nudged Dave and whispered that it was time to take his medicine. I thought for sure he'd be wobbly, so I offered to help him. Nope. He was fine. He grabbed his phone and his water and headed to the bathroom, only six steps away. Out of habit, he closed the door so the light wouldn't disturb me. I felt relieved at the way he trotted off to the bathroom so full of energy. Being exhausted myself, I rolled onto my side, took a deep breath, and attempted to relax and go back to sleep.

A moment later I heard something fall. I perched in bed . . . rigid . . . listening. I'm constantly nagging him, so I refrained from heading to the bathroom door to check on him. I just waited. Then . . . another sound of something small dropping . . . then CLUNK. I knew it was the sound of his body hitting the floor. *Damnit!*

I flew into the bathroom, my legs not moving as fast as I wanted them to, and when I got there I found Dave on the floor. He was lying on his left side, the toilet seat appeared to be broken, and there was blood on the floor. The twenty-five years I spent as a first responder should have prepared me for moments like this: First step, assess his level of consciousness and breathing; second step, find out what's bleeding; third step, check for any additional injuries; last step, attempt to get him up. Hospice said to call them before attempting to lift him, but I was not going to have Dave lie on the floor all that time.

I knew what had happened based on his nightly rituals and the scene around me. Dave's nose hole requires constant maintenance. When he gets up during the night to use the bathroom, he often grabs his little flashlight and looks in the mirror to see whether his face needs any tending to. Last night he dropped something on the floor while performing this task. While attempting to pick it up, his momentum continued forward as his left leg collapsed under him. I wasn't sure whether he'd hit his head on the porcelain of the toilet, but it seemed that as he went down, he instinctively wrapped his arms around his head. I think his left elbow bumped the toilet seat, knocking one of the hinges off as he went down. His paper-thin skin was slightly torn on that elbow, which was causing a bit of bleeding. Physically, he was in relatively decent shape.

As I helped him up, he said his legs felt like spaghetti. After standing, he attempted to take a step. As he started to go down, I wrapped my arms around his belly from behind him and prevented the fall. I perched him against the vanity and ran for that little bench we have in the office. I scooted it under his bottom so he could sit. There he sat for the next fifteen minutes, breathing like he had run a marathon and wondering why his legs had betrayed him. He sat on the bench with his elbows on the vanity, his head in his hands, and the mirror in front of him. I knew he was badly shaken. I imagine he was wondering just how bad this was going to get. I think he might be getting to the point of wanting it all to be over.

I called the after-hours number for hospice and waited about ten minutes for the evening nurse to call me back. She's the same one who came to our house last week, our third nurse. I recited everything that's been transpiring since

Monday evening, much the way I've been reciting Dave's condition to our doctors for the last three years. I told her about my concern over Dave's recent tremors.

"Have you changed medications in the last couple days?" she asked.

"We added ibuprofen, but that's it," I replied.

She responded, "Often, the only other reason for tremors is a gradual decline towards end-of-life."

BAM! The roller coaster hit rock bottom.

The nurse said she would be at our house in forty-five to fifty minutes. I turned on the outside lights for her and unlocked the front door. Apparently Dave decided the best way to get back in bed was to crawl. Probably not a bad idea.

With Dave back in bed, I sat on the edge next to him, weighing in my mind whether to tell him that the nurse said the tremors are likely an indication of his body declining. Yes. I knew he'd want to know.

After I told him, I swear he was ready to close his eyes and stop breathing right there and then. I said to myself, "No! Not yet! You're declining . . . you're not dying tonight!" I crawled up onto the bed and into his arms, then cried and cried and cried. I know it hurts him to see me like this. I racked my brain to remember whether there's anything else I need to tell him before he goes. Is there something else I need to say?

"This has been a really rough road," I squeaked out through tears.

"And I wouldn't want anyone but you in the driver's seat," he said.

While waiting for the nurse, I contemplated recording the next forty-five minutes on tape. Dave was not dying tonight, but our conversation was as if he had been. I'll never be able to remember everything he said, and I'm going to want to hear all the wonderful things he told me over and over and over after he's no longer here. But I didn't record anything. Other than what is written here, his words from this night will remain a mystery. I don't remember anything he said.

Dave's clarity of thought is remarkable. His brain seems to be functioning optimally, clearer than since all the drugs began.

He asked if I would get his laptop and bring it to him. In the twenty-one years we've been married, Dave has never wanted his computer in bed. He unfolded it and opened a Word document. I may have earned the nickname Snoop Dog over the years, but I really do try to honor his privacy. I told him I wasn't looking, but I figured whatever he was doing must have been important.

"That's okay," he said when he noticed me looking, "I'm printing it out for you."

"Is that my letter?" I asked.

"Yes. It's not finished," he replied.

At least six months ago, maybe more, I asked Dave to write me a love letter. Why in the world would I need a love letter? I have every greeting card this man has ever given me expressing his love. Months passed before I asked him if he'd written my letter.

"What letter?" he asks.

"My love letter," I say. I feel I'm being petty by reminding him.

He writes on the top of a piece of paper, "Patty's letter." It's at the top of his to-do list. Eventually he writes other things on the list. They get crossed off as they get accomplished, and the list disappears.

I wrestle in my brain, "He must have written the letter if he threw away the list. He wouldn't have gotten rid of the list if there was still something left to do on it."

For the next few months, in the back of my mind, I won-
der if this letter is folded in thirds, slipped in an envelope,
and tucked in a drawer, only to be found by me when he's
no longer here. I refuse to ask him. I tell myself not to be
disappointed if I never find a letter. I know he loves me.
Really, what else does he have to say?

"When did you start the letter?" I asked.

"Sometime around September," he replied.

I imagine it must have been around the time we stopped treatment and started hospice.

"It was hard to go back to," he added. "It's not finished because I never gave up."

Sitting on the bed with him, I saw the top of the letter on his computer screen: "My Dearest Patty." I heard the printer in the other room buzzing. Reminding him he's not dying tonight, I told him, "You can finish the letter tomorrow." I regretted my words almost immediately. He hadn't finished the letter because he'd never given up; therefore, this probably should remain an unfinished letter.

"You're the only reason I've stuck around this long," he told me. He loves his Snookums.

When the nurse arrived, she checked Dave quickly and left soon after. Thank God he wasn't badly hurt in the fall.

It was 4 a.m. when she left. I snuggled as close to Dave as I could. Even Sadie joined us on the bed, a rare treat. We have the most unusual dog. Although I've trained all my dogs to only jump on the bed when offered, she rarely joins us; she usually just looks at us as we pat the bed and call her name, then walks away to lie someplace else. We always get a chuckle out of her quirkiness. Dave slipped into slumber easily. I barely grazed the surface of sleep. I got up shortly before 8 a.m.

The roller coaster is whizzing along on even ground again. He's still here.

There's a little mantra I've been repeating to myself over the last three years. When I find myself getting overly anxious about losing Dave, I say, "He's here today, he'll probably be here tomorrow, and more than likely the day after that." The thought of having three days has been enough to calm me down. But I know there will come a time when I can only say, "He's here today . . ."

Jessica came to visit us today. She spent about an hour speaking with us about the events that have unfolded since the last time she saw Dave. She ordered all the pharmaceuticals we need, then picked up her bags to leave. I walked her out of the bedroom to the front door, asking her, "Are these latest changes signs of decline?"

"Probably," she replied.

The roller coaster shifted from even ground to a sudden stomach-lurching drop . . . again.

After she left, I lay on the bed next to Dave. I placed a pillow across his legs so I could lie across him; it was too uncomfortable for both of us to lie on his bony body.

He asked me if we'd gotten the camper back yet. It's been at the shop for a warranty issue and is then going directly to the body shop for collision work. When I told him we still don't have it back yet, he asked, "Who are we going to get to camp with you?" My Dave . . . always concerned about me.

"There's no one I like enough, other than you, to spend several days with in a one-hundred-square-foot tin can," I replied.

He chuckled, probably because he's the one who usually refers to the camper as a tin can. Or maybe it was because he knew I was telling the truth.

"You're my only camping partner. If I camp with anyone in the future, they will be supplying their own camper or tent," I added.

He knew I wasn't kidding.

Dave has often said I should get myself a little teardrop camper. I know nothing about campers, but the idea of not sleeping on the ground anymore in my three-person tent with my bad back does have some appeal.

The pandemic hits, then we climb aboard the cancer train, and life as we know it changes.

Dave is being checked in for his first set of scans at the hospital. He'll be a couple of hours, so I take a stab at Googling RVs to keep myself busy. There's so much to learn, but I foresee I'll be spending a lot of time in hospitals and will need to focus my brain on something other than cancer.

I decide on a ten- to twelve-foot travel trailer that can be pulled by my SUV. When Dave is done with his scans, I tell him of my brief research. It looks like I can buy a little camper for about $10,000. He gives me two thumbs up!

As I dive deep into my research of campers, I start to wonder whether I should get something a little bigger because Dave might travel with me. "Dave," I ask, "can you see yourself traveling via travel trailer? Not camping, per se, but I'm wondering with COVID and your immune system if you'll travel with me. If so, I'm going to need to get a camper bigger than a teardrop; we're going to need a couple's camper."

Dave gives me an affirmative response, and that's all I need to run with.

Having a reputation for over-researching everything, I don't disappoint and research the hell out of the camper. I select a twenty-four-foot travel trailer. It's the perfect size for us and has all the bells and whistles! But it turns out I'll need a pickup truck to pull a camper of this size, so the search for a solid, preowned truck ensues. Terms such as "payload," "GVWR," "CCC," and "UVW" are becoming part of my daily vernacular.

Dave is still in the recovery room when I tell him I bought a truck. With the cost of everything climbing quickly during COVID, I'm excited that I bought my first truck for under $30,000. Actually, I haven't purchased it yet, but I did find it and scheduled a test drive, and that's almost as good as pulling the trigger. Later, after he wakes up from the next surgery, I tell him I couldn't find the camper I was looking for on an RV lot, so I'd custom-ordered a brand new one from the dealer—which cost about the same as the truck.

Dave is getting immunotherapy every three weeks, but there's an option to get a double dose every six weeks, so I plan a five-week bucket-list trip, which we're calling "BLT 2023," so we can be home in time for treatment. We plan to visit Arizona, Montana, Utah, and South Dakota. Coming from the East Coast of North Carolina, it will be an interesting trip to connect the dots.

We pull out of our street with plans to be on the road for thirty-five days, drive about seven thousand miles, and set up camp eighteen times. I'm ready to do it all; I want Dave to help only as much as he's comfortable doing.

We have a fabulous trip! We make impromptu stops, take lots of pictures, see everything we want to see, and thoroughly enjoy each other's company. Naturally, we have a couple of hiccups along the way, but we tackle everything as a team.

I read a Facebook post I made in my camper group after a particularly harrowing experience. My last sentence is, "As I said yesterday, stuff is stuff, people are people. Dave is my person and man . . . we killed it today!" That, in a nutshell, is the entire flavor of the trip. I blog about it on

Facebook, and Dave keeps his own journal. Adding his humor, he emails his journal to at least twenty people who anxiously wait for weekly installments.

Dave, who has always had a charming ability to embellish life's experiences, still revels in telling the story of how his wife told him she had bought a new truck, then a new RV, when he was coming out of anesthesia following a surgery. He also loves to tease me that I ended up spending six times my initial estimate. But it turned out to be a wonderful investment by giving us priceless memories.

While I was thinking about this, my eyes wandered back to the letter Dave wrote, which was still sitting on the printer. He must be amazed that Snoop Dog hasn't read it yet. I'm not ready to read it.

The roller coaster is chugging along on another slow climb of uncertainty, but today is the day the scale tilted. Dave spent more time in bed than out of bed. It's the first day that the bed didn't get made up like it always has in the past, with the decorative pillows, a stuffed gingerbread man (my spirit animal) on my side, and a sloth (Dave's spirit animal) on his.

13

Thursday, October 19

*T*he roller coaster is screaming downward. This must be the final descent.

Yesterday afternoon I pulled the letter off the printer. It was typical Dave: caring, loving, and with a bit of humor. He wishes he'd started the letter sooner so it could have been handwritten. He said letters of this sort are supposed to be penned, not typed. I told him I loved it, and he said something about "true literary gifts being rewritten, not just written." He apologized for not giving it several rewrites. I know in my heart there is nothing left for either of us to say.

Dave has been unable to maneuver around the house without me since the fall. His legs are buckling, and he's extremely wobbly. I plead with him to never walk anywhere without me. If he falls and breaks a hip, he will need to be transported to the hospice center where he will spend his remaining days. We cannot let that happen.

I always put Dave on my right side to help him maneuver about the house. We each wrap an arm around the other, face forward, and call cadence: right, left, right, left, right . . . this is my rifle, this is my gun, one is for fighting, one is for fun . . . sound off . . . now walk like a crab . . . to the side . . . to the side. There tends to be a fair amount of laughter at our clumsy attempt to move around. We resemble a pinball bouncing off the hallway walls. The laughter feels as good as the tears feel bad.

It was almost a normal night except that Dave has lost all interest in food. I read the pamphlet that hospice provided. The lack of interest in food is a normal sign of something referred to as "transitioning"—transitioning from a living body to a dying one, from a physical being to a spiritual being. It's a process.

We watched TV while Dave ate his slushie and we snuggled on the couch. His slushie is a concoction I've invented of Italian ice blended with pineapple–orange juice, so it's loose and slushy. Something about the cold and the texture appeals to him. He says he looks forward to slushie time all day! Between the slushies and the pineapple–mango smoothies from our favorite coffee shop that he's been drinking almost every morning since hospice started, Dave seems to have a new affinity for pineapple. Much the way he has no sense of smell, he also has no sense of taste, but he knows what pineapple used to taste like so he eats with his memory. Dave liked pineapple when he was healthy, but the only time I ever remember him commenting about it was when he would refer to the pineapple that was available to us on our trip to Hawaii. "That . . . was the perfect pineapple," he had said.

When we got into bed, Dave again asked me to bring him his computer. While he scrolled through the New York Post website, I continued to kid myself that because of his interest in outside events, he's not stepping closer to another stage of transitioning: withdrawal. He opened his bank's website and said, "I'm transferring some money to our joint account from my slush account. It's for the kids when they come up for the funeral."

"Okay," I said.

"Offer it to them," he responded. "If they want it, fine. If they don't, that's fine too. But this will help prevent causing hardship for them." Then he asked me, "When you die, you'll take care of my kids, right?"

I was shocked by this question. He knows my will names his three children, who at this point are all in their forties and are professionals with PhDs, as my heirs. But I replied, "Of course I will."

"By the time you sell the house, it could be worth a million dollars . . . just take care of them," he pressed.

I'm hurt that he thinks there's a chance I would do something else with my estate. I reassured him that I will make sure his kids receive my estate upon my death.

After I got ready for bed, I did all the final checks of the evening, including getting Dave's middle-of-the-night meds ready and checking that his urinal jug was waiting for him on his nightstand. We've started putting one there since the day after he fell. It seems to be a good solution. Dave is able to stand, lean against the bed for support, pee in the jug, and leave it for me to empty. I put away his computer and we snuggled before turning out the light.

Speaking has become very difficult for Dave, especially during the night when his mouth is extremely dry. This awful tumor has been growing so rapidly. It's growing into his lip and onto the roof of his mouth and causes him extreme pain.

At about 3:30 in the morning, I woke abruptly because I felt Dave's body jerk. When I asked him if he was okay, he mumbled, "Get me to the bathroom."

I assumed he needed to sit on the toilet, so I jumped out of my side of the bed, ran around to him, and embraced him from the front, knowing we would never fit through the doorway side by side. We did a rather humorous two-step to get into the bathroom. Turns out he needed to vomit in the sink. The liquid that poured out of him was dark brown, nearly black. I held him as he continued to wretch. It seemed to be never-ending.

Dave hates to vomit. No one really likes to vomit, but Dave really hates it.

As I held onto him so he wouldn't fall, I realized jumping up so quickly had made me lightheaded and given me a nauseous stomach. What a pair we were! I pulled the little bench over and lowered Dave to the seat before I went to lie on the bed. It took me only a few minutes to recover. I only wish it were that easy for Dave.

Like last night, Dave sat on the stool, elbows on the vanity, head in hands, looking down. I didn't know what was going on in his head. I imagined fear was at the top of the list, but knowing Dave, this probably has more to do with him feeling bad for me than feeling bad for himself. He must be wondering how long this is going to go on.

Dave sat there for a while before he was ready for me to help him get back into bed and lose himself in sleep. I lay beside him, but I didn't sleep. My mind kept bouncing from topic to topic like a house fly at a summer barbeque. Ultimately, I got out of bed around 5:30 a.m., knowing the chance for sleep had passed. I'm starting to wonder how many more nights I can do this. How many more nights can Dave do this?

Today was the first day of early voting in our municipal election. As usual, Dave is more well-informed on political candidates than 98 percent of the general public. And I'm a strong believer in paying attention to your local election, as that's the one that affects you directly. Dave and I were supposed to go to the Board of Elections today to vote, but that didn't happen. So Dave asked me to make sure I vote and to get him an absentee ballot. I wasn't thrilled about leaving him alone, but he promised he wouldn't move from the bed. So I drove the forty-five minutes to vote and hand in the request for an absentee ballot for Dave. The clerk couldn't hand me a ballot. He said it had to be mailed to the address of the registered voter. When I asked him how quickly it would be mailed, he said by tomorrow.

When I returned home, it was 3:30 in the afternoon, and Dave hadn't left the bed. He hasn't left the bed all day. I asked him what he wanted.

"I want to go to sleep and not wake up."

My heart could not possibly break any more than it did right then.

"The nurse is scheduled to come tomorrow," I told him. "We can discuss a higher level of sedation so you can sleep more . . . unless you want me to have a nurse come today?"

"Tomorrow is fine," he said.

I am absolutely panicked! I'm only going to have Dave to talk to for another day. I have imagined going into this moment dozens of times, yet I am definitely not ready for it.

Dave's wish to go to sleep and not wake up made me think of the little blue pamphlet from hospice. This is more transitioning. This means we're getting closer to the end. I've run through a checklist in my mind:

- Withdrawal—he's said he's done with visitors. Weeks ago we also discussed whether he wants to be surrounded by family during his last days. Nope. Just me.
- Sleep—he's sleeping more and wants to sleep even more.
- Disorientation—he seems to have one foot in another world. He's not on high doses of medication, yet he's seeing things and has started talking out loud to invisible people. They're often people we know, sometimes not. They're kind of like dreams, but he's not asleep. Oddly enough, he's aware when this happens and will say, "Did you see that? I must have been in my other world."
- Food—he has lost all interest.

Sadie is really out of sorts. I took her for a walk this morning. She has spent the entire day alone in the basement on the landing. I can't believe it's really going to be just the two of us soon. I can't help but think after Dave dies: First there will be all the formalities—the funeral, the memorial service, the repast at our house. Then everyone will go home. It will be Sadie and me. Just us.

What a shock! At 4:30 p.m., Dave wanted to get up, go to the bathroom, get cleaned up, and walk around the house. Go Dave! My rollercoaster is cruising upward again.

14

Friday, October 20

J've started getting in some extra snuggle time with Dave while we're still on the couch before jumping up for the nighttime routine. We had a great night last night watching TV and snuggling. I turned to him so we were face-to-face, and I lay across his lap, carefully wedging a throw pillow somewhere so Dave's boniness wouldn't poke me. He willingly wrapped his arms around me.

"You deserve a lot of love," Dave said.

That's one of the sweetest things I've ever heard someone say in my life. I replied, "But you won't be here to give me that love."

He answered, "There are many kinds of love."

I smiled and nodded.

As tired as I am after four nights of practically no sleep, I almost dread sleep. I lose all those hours of being with Dave. Last night we both slept well. That was good for both of us. As usual, I woke up before he did. I wonder whether he will change his mind about wanting to be asleep more.

When Dave woke up, he said, "I don't want to get out of bed anymore."

"You don't have to," I said.

I reached out to Bobby, our friend and pastor, last night and asked him to drop by today. He really is our friend first, then our pastor. Over the last few years, the three of us have been discussing "check-out day." Once Bobby arrived, he followed me to the bedroom. I plopped down on the bed next to Dave, in my spot, while Dave and Bobby said hello and shook hands. Bobby's demeanor is always outgoing and friendly. He sat on the little bench that's been making its way around the house lately.

"I think check-out time is coming soon," Dave said.

Bobby subtly smiled when Dave said those words. So honest. So raw. So Dave. He appears so unafraid.

"Ah, check-out day," Bobby said. "That means check-in day is coming."

We continued to chat and share stories, then finally we prayed. That's when I always cry. There's something about listening to someone else's words to God that always makes me cry. I'm not convinced there is a God, but I'm not convinced there's not.

Before Bobby left, Dave said to him, "I need you to watch out for my best buddy" while patting me on the leg.

Bobby assured him, "You are both woven into the community. Patty will be cared for after you are no longer here."

The next visitor today was Jessica. I filled her in on Dave's decision not to leave the bed anymore, so we headed to the bedroom. Jessica was her cheery self and was met by Dave being his charming self. After the pleasantries, we got to the meat of why she was here today. I asked Dave to speak. This was too important to come from me.

He explained that he's tired of taking pills, he's tired of being tired, he's tired of doing this and doesn't want to anymore. We talked about adding a medication for anxiety, part of that "comfort pack" hospice gave us early on. She told me it will help Dave relax and sleep more and that the shift towards comfort over alertness will be gradual.

When Jessica left, Dave said he was willing to try a pineapple-mango smoothie from our favorite coffee shop. Although these smoothies have been a staple for nearly a month now, I'm surprised he showed interest today. I drove five minutes to pick it up and changed my usual order to decaf espresso. I know I've been taking in too much caffeine lately, and the last thing I need is the jitters or more sleeplessness. The baristas, all adoring fans of Dave's, wrote loving, encouraging messages on our cold cups.

Ultimately, Dave had little interest in the smoothie, but he wanted to sit on the side of the bed and have me go through his dresser drawers while he directed me what to do with specific items.

"Are you doing this for me?" I asked.

"No . . . yes . . . well . . . I'm doing this for me too," he replied.

I'm fairly certain he was doing it more for me than for him. Dave is continuing to take care of me.

He took his pain meds and his new anxiety med, lorazepam, at 3 p.m. Normally he sleeps for about three hours that time of day; after that, I wake him or he won't be able to sleep later in the night. Today he slept for four hours. I checked on him for the last hour and he seemed unwakable. I realized there was no reason to wake him. This is what he wants; to sleep more . . . to continue to transition. So I sat in the living room getting some work done on the computer.

Dave wrote his own obituary a month ago so I wouldn't have to. After he emailed it to me, he told me to change anything I saw that needed changing. I wasn't surprised that it was perfect. It was fact-based but with a bit of humor thrown in. Dave has always liked journalism. It seems appropriate he gets to write this.

I want to write an addendum to the obituary to post on his Facebook page and on the funeral home's website when the time comes. I will ask him to read it to make sure he approves. What a strange existence we're now living.

I started writing, "And now a note from Patty . . ." I sat looking at our comfy, beautiful beach house that I've wanted most of my life, our place to retire and make all our dreams come true. I could hear Dave breathing from all the way down the hall. I wonder how many days it will be before I sit here and no longer hear his breath. The fear of losing him is growing. "He's here today, he'll probably be here tomorrow, and more than likely the day after that," I keep reciting to myself.

When Dave finally woke from his nap, we spent a few hours together. The lorazepam, which is often used to treat anxiety, is supposed to relax his muscles and his mind to help him sleep. Just to be clear, Dave has not exhibited any signs of anxiety. He's certainly less anxious than me. But not only did Dave feel completely knocked on his ass when he woke up but the little "imaginary" visualizations he's been having have become full-on hallucinations. I've finally realized they are not from the medication. He has one foot in this world and his other foot somewhere else. That's exactly how Dave described it once.

I'm not going to lie. They are a little funny, but they are also a little scary. Knowing he's so far away from me now is the start of my knowing he won't be here forever.

While getting ready for bed tonight, I heard Dave say something, but I couldn't understand what. "What, Bumpy?" I called out. I don't remember how long I've been calling Dave that, but it's been nearly as long as we've been married.

"I was talking to the captain," he answered.

"Talking to the captain about what?"

"The submarine."

"Oh, of course, the submarine." I chuckled as this seemed perfectly reasonable to him.

Dave wanted to get up and walk around the house tonight. Out to the front door we went, holding each other like conjoined twins, walking into the kitchen, then back to the bedroom.

He wanted to go to the bathroom and look at himself. He's appalled at the physical changes of his face. He thinks he's ugly. It's so painful to me that he sees just the anatomical changes to his face. I see only the gold that's inside him.

15

Saturday, October 21

*L*ast night was bearable. We woke up at 3 a.m. because Dave had to pee. He sleeps so soundly now; he never moves in his sleep. The minute he does, I know something is happening. As he settled back to sleep, he mumbled to himself, or maybe he was mumbling to me.

"We shouldn't go to Niagara Falls," he said. "We should go straight home since we don't have enough cold medicine."

"Okay, we'll go straight home," I replied.

Dave drifted back to sleep, occasionally twitching, jerking, and muttering. I lay there until nearly 5 a.m., wishing for sleep. Eventually, I drifted off for about an hour and a half and had a series of short nightmares, barely waking between each one. My brain serves me well by not letting me remember them when I wake for the day. Now I know that even sleep is not a place I can escape.

I started my morning routine—bathroom, coffee, feed Sadie, open the laptop—and was overcome with raw emotion. I cried. I cried hard. I cried hard enough I was afraid I'd wake Dave even though I was several rooms away.

This has officially become unbearable.

I will be forever changed.

No amount of mental preparation can prepare you to watch the person you love with all your soul deteriorate.

I thought I heard Dave stir, so I wiped my eyes and trotted down the hall. Standing over him, I waited for movement. Nothing. I sat on the side of the bed and gently traced his face, his ears, the top of his head. He hasn't shaved in days and his whiskers are soft. I like the way they feel. Looking at my hand, I noticed my beautiful engagement ring and wedding band.

It's funny that Dave thought our night of passion in Jamaica had been a one-time thing. Based on the way I kept my distance for so many years, what could he think? But I knew otherwise.

About six or seven months after we'd returned from Jamaica, I drove to a wonderful department store in New Jersey that had a gigantic jewelry section.

I head straight for the wedding rings. I tell the gal I'm looking for a diamond ring . . . an engagement ring. I've done my research about the three C's—color, cut, and clarity—and I want a classic, round stone. Quality is far more important to me than size.

She shows me a gorgeous stone! It glistens in the bright lights of the store. Wanting a proper setting to showcase such a beautiful diamond, I look for a yellow-gold band with two stones of descending size on the left and two on the right in a white gold setting. We find the perfect one. I slide the band on my left ring finger, and the salesperson uses tweezers to drop the showstopper in the setting. It's perfect! I can visualize wearing it for the rest of my life. She writes all the details about the setting and the stone on the back of her business card and hands it to me.

The next time I see Dave, I coyly pull out the business card and hand it to him. He looks at it and flips it over, not sure what the gibberish written on the back is supposed to mean. "This is what you're going to need when you decide to ask me to marry you," I say.

Unbeknownst to me, Dave wastes no time. The following weekend he drives to the store and buys the ring.

When Dave woke up, I asked him if he was okay. I have difficulty understanding his words when he first wakes up and am starting to wonder whether I should keep a recorder or my phone close by. What if I can't understand his final words? I need to have them on tape so I can share them and decipher what he said.

We talked about the new drug and how it makes him feel. I secretly wish he weren't taking it because it steals my time with him. But the drug puts him in a place he wants to be, one of comfort and sleep. This is where true love is defined. This is where I give up my moments of Dave time so that he is content. The moments we do have, while he is alert, are even more valuable now.

He wanted to do his morning routine. He's become incredibly tolerant of allowing me to assist him with his movement. I helped him to the bathroom sink, where he leaned against the vanity for stability while I placed behind him the metal stool we've been using in the shower. I sat on the stool and placed my hands on his hips and my forehead on the small of his back. I ingrained the moment into my brain . . . the feel of his hips, the way the curve of his back fits my head . . .

He asked me if he should shave, and I asked him if he wanted to. I know this is painful for him, as the skin on the right side of his face is so tender with the growing tumor. I peeked around his waist, rested my chin on his hip bone, and watched him shave. The whiskers were long on his chin, and he scraped three times with the razor, still not removing the hair.

"You need a new razor," I said as I offered him one from the drawer. Still holding his hips, I moved my chin to rest on the other side of his waist.

"I don't want you to remember me like this," he said.

"Like what?" I asked, feigning naivety.

"Like this," he said while motioning to his weak body and his disfigured face.

"How 'bout if I remember you getting ready for your Saturday morning flying lessons in Spring Lake?" I asked.

He nodded. He was still shaving, and it's getting too painful for him to smile, but he liked that idea. Seeing his agreement, I continued, "Or how about when I would wait to meet you on Friday nights down the shore so we could start our weekends at our happy place?"

In 2007, after we buy our little 910-square-foot beach condo in Spring Lake, every weekend becomes a mini vacation. Dave and I have some of our best memories there. On Fridays in the summer, I use personal time to leave work by noon. I zip home, change clothes, grab some perishables out of the fridge, throw them in the cooler, and call the dog . . . or dogs. We jump in the car and head south for seventy-five miles until we get to our happy place at the Jersey Shore.

Dave is certainly not getting out of work early and, coming from New York, always hits more traffic than me. By the time he arrives around 7 p.m., I've already enjoyed the relaxing atmosphere of coastal living for a solid four hours. Dave is still wound tight from a traffic-filled ride, complete with all the idiots and road rage that accompany a trip southbound on the Garden State Parkway on a Friday afternoon in the summer.

We are both starving and usually decide dinner at St. Stephens is on the agenda. It's right down the street from us, and anyplace we can walk to is a bonus, knowing cocktails will be ordered the moment we walk in the door. Dave orders me a Captain and Diet Coke and himself a Tanqueray Gin & Tonic. The weekend officially begins, and Dave already looks forward to tomorrow morning's flight lesson.

Dave liked the idea of being remembered like that. We racked our brains to think of the other restaurants we liked in Spring Lake. It seems so long ago.

I continued to watch him shave. It reminded me of the times I used to watch my dad shave when I was a child. I'd sit on the toilet with my ankles crossed and my legs swinging and watch him standing there in his tighty-whities with his white undershirt tucked in. Dave tucks in his undershirt the same way.

Eventually he was ready for his shower, so I moved the stool back into the shower stall. I helped Dave step in and assisted him with getting seated, then left the bathroom to give him some privacy. I waited just outside the bathroom door, as Dave can no longer shout very loud when he's done. As I helped him get dry and dressed, he told me who he was willing to see today. First he mentions Jeremy, the owner of our favorite coffee shop.

When Dave and I retire in 2015, he moves to our retirement home in North Carolina a month before I do. Having a whole lot of time on his hands and being in a new state, he pokes around town, investigating new places. One of the places he stumbles upon is The Daily Grind, a coffee and ice cream shop with a beach vibe. The owners are Jeremy and Tracey. Jeremy is there most days and is more a mix of Monty Hall and a used car salesman than a laid-back coffee-shop owner, but he has a flair for remembering names, introducing people, and making them feel comfortable.

By the time I join Dave in North Carolina, he's ready to introduce me to the coffee shop and its patrons. Upon meeting Jeremy, I'm a little overwhelmed by his overbearing personality, but I like the coffee shop.

We stop in from time to time and eventually become part of the "retiree coffee klatch." We all sit in a second room, painted purple and off to the side where there's no secret handshake to enter, but it's clear you need to be one of the gang. The retirees talk about retired people stuff: fixed incomes, tourists, grandchildren, recently developed aches and pains. Since I retired at the age of fifty, it takes me a little longer to find common ground, but Dave is a natural with any age group.

It is in this coffee shop that we meet Pastor Bobby. Bobby is sitting at his table and us at ours. We strike up a conversation. I'm quite surprised when I find out Bobby has dedicated his life to spreading the word of Jesus; he doesn't look or sound like a pastor. I enjoy our conversation that day and will be fortunate to bump into Bobby many times over the years. Bobby believes everything happens for a reason; I believe meeting Bobby is just a chance meeting.

Over the next eight years, Jeremy and Tracey become two of our dearest friends. We vacation with them and dine and party at their home more times than we can count. They have more friends than anyone I've ever known, but we become part of their inner circle and they a part of ours.

As years go by, Jeremy and Tracey, talented entrepreneurs, move their coffee shop to a bigger, more beautiful location. They attach a wine bar and hire more staff. All their employees are friends or family of friends. No one gets a job here by anonymously putting in an application; you must be connected. THE coffee shop, as we call it even though there are a half dozen other coffee shops on the island, becomes our hangout, and the baristas become our extended family.

Dave becomes the only member of the Free Coffee for Life Club, a club that doesn't really exist but is a euphemism because there's never a charge for Dave's coffee. Dave, having the wonderful and captivating personality he has, engages all the lovely ladies with his sincere interest in their lives. He remembers who goes to school where, who has a volleyball game, whose sister is coming to visit, and what college they're applying to. I must admit, this is not an area I excel in, but Dave is a natural, and all the girls love my harmless husband. Even Colonel Tom says, "Walking into the coffee shop with Dave is like walking in with a rock star."

As Dave's illness progresses, the girls replace Dave's favorite coffee and half-and-half with pineapple–mango smoothies and often hand-deliver them to our home. Jeremy and Tracey offer anything they can do to make our lives easier.

One day, Tracey calls me to say, "I know how you like your flower garden a certain way, and I imagine you haven't had time to garden. Can I send over my guys to pull weeds?" I don't take her up on it, but I'm astounded at the love our friends feel for us.

One of Jeremy's most endearing and simultaneously annoying traits is his physically affectionate behavior towards everyone. He has become like a brother to me and often greets me with, "You look gorgeous today!" followed by a kiss half on the lips/half on the cheek and a hug. Twenty years younger than Dave, Jeremy thoroughly enjoys creating playful discomfort with all his older male friends when he climbs all over them with hugs and kisses. Usually, Dave says something like, "Get off of me, you ass-hole." This is always a laugh for all of us and quite the normal greeting for these two.

Dave said that along with seeing Jeremy, he'd like to see two of his favorite baristas, Ashley and Jaiden. These ladies are more than just coffee servers; they are friends and the people Dave is choosing to see during his last days.

He told me to give everyone five minutes, which really meant ten or fifteen. He also asked me to let them know he wouldn't have his manhole cover on and that it was okay if they didn't want to come; he would understand. He knows it's difficult to look at his face, and it's been getting more difficult by the day as the tumor grows, especially for someone who's never seen the inside of a nose hole.

The decision was not a difficult one. They both replied "Yes!" to my text, and Jaiden asked, "When can I come?" Jaiden is only seventeen years old but is wise beyond her years.

Each of the visits was short and sweet. I brought each visi-tor to the bedroom, starting with Jeremy. I hopped on the bed to Dave's right, where I always sit, and offered Jeremy the lit-tle bench seat that Pastor Bobby sat in. Dave had a fair amount of medication in him and was having difficulty staying in the moment, but he managed to converse with Jeremy. Jeremy was outgoing and gregarious, as that's how he's most comfortable being. It wasn't until he neared the end of his visit that he became emotional. He mentioned that he doesn't cry and that this is difficult for him. I know exactly what he means. There was a time I didn't cry either. Now I cry all the time. Well, I try not to cry too much in front of Dave.

Jeremy's eyes were red and teary when he said, "You know I love you . . . right?"

Dave didn't respond.

Jeremy repeated himself: "You know I love you, right Dave? I do, you know."

As the emotional tension built in the room, Dave peeled back the covers and nodded towards his manhood with the implication Jeremy take care of his needs. Jeremy burst out laughing, and the tension in the room was eased. Jeremy gently hugged and kissed Dave, then left when his ten minutes were over.

Next came Ashley, followed by Jaiden. Dave continued to make people feel special because that's what he does. He engaged the ladies with questions about their lives. With Dave, it's never just about him. I remained on the bed while they chatted, always ready to quietly signal when it was time for them to leave should Dave show signs he needed to rest or it was getting too painful for him to speak. I know the girls felt special that they had this time with Dave. And then, Dave slept.

He slept at least five hours this afternoon. Other than going out in the yard for a moment with Sadie, I was afraid to leave the house. I feared being away for any period of time in case Dave needed something. I spent time on my computer, feeling sorry for both of us. And I baked chocolate chip cookies for dinner.

Dave's sisters and children periodically checked in with me via text to ask how Dave was doing. Except Megan. Megan checks in daily. I've been truthful with everyone, but I've also been a little bit vague.

After checking on Dave at around 5:30 p.m., his normal time to wake from a nap, I sat on the edge of the bed while he slept. He was sleeping so deeply that I took his hand and touched his face without waking him. There was a little gnat flying around his face and it landed on his left eyelid. I tried to shoo it away and accidentally flicked Dave's face. His eyes fluttered open and I apologized.

I asked him if he needed a drink, and he nodded. I rushed to get some pineapple juice with an elbow straw, like my mother used to give me when I was sick. He sipped the juice while lying down. Since his mouth is so dry, his words are not audible unless he drinks first. I set the juice on the nightstand. Dave was still lying on his back with both hands on his chest as I took his hands in mine and rested my forehead on them.

He very clearly said, "I'm so lucky to have you." I repeated the same words back to him, as my feelings are the same.

Eventually, Dave rose so he could pee, still using the little jug on the nightstand. I left the room for a moment because this is one of the times he likes just a little privacy. He stood with the back of his thighs leaning against the bed for support, but I worried he might tip over so I quietly stood in the doorway to the hall, wondering whether I was close enough to sprint across the room and around the bed if his legs buckled. Probably not.

I asked Dave if he'd like to take a hot bath. Our days of "Tub Talks" are over. I'm so glad I will have those memories of our tubs together. I'm already savoring them.

Then Dave proclaimed, "Tonight, I want to watch a movie." I shook my head in disbelief at the normalcy of that statement.

Dave enjoyed his hot tub. When he was done, I went into the bathroom to help him up and out of the tub, then into the bedroom to dry and dress in clean clothes for bed. We two-stepped out into the living room, still bouncing like a pinball in the hallway. I handed him the remote control and made his pineapple–mango slushie, which he requested. I made it thinner than the smoothies, stressing over whether I should. *Don't sweat the small shit . . . and it's all small shit!* I heard in my head. These words have become Dave's mantra over the last month, and he reminds me of them regularly.

I delivered the slushie to Dave, and as I returned to the kitchen, he let out an exclamation. I looked over to see him standing with the slushie cup, the slushie dumped across the sofa. My biggest fear was that he was standing between the sofa and the coffee table with nothing to grab hold of. He looked helpless, and all I cared about was getting him safe and dry. I scurried around, cleaning him up first, then the sofa, so we could get to where we'd been ten minutes before.

I asked him if he wanted another slushie, hoping he would even though I knew the answer. No. He didn't. His diet for the day consisted of less than half of a fruit smoothie that Jeremy brought this morning.

Nothing seemed worthwhile on television, so I suggested we watch a movie we've both seen many times. We watched *The Accountant* with Ben Affleck. I periodically took peeks at Dave, who was sitting to my left as he usually is when we sit on the couch together. I often saw his eyes roll up under his eyelids. He seemed to be going in and out of this world. More transitioning. I guess he never really saw the movie, but at least I got to snuggle up next to him.

I could barely keep my eyes open and was completely exhausted. When it was time for bed, Dave sat on the sofa, scrolling through his phone while I performed the usual night-time routine of brushing my teeth, opening the bed, letting the dog out, and getting the middle-of-the-night meds ready. It was only then that I took my position next to him as we two-stepped across the living room to head towards the bedroom.

He stopped short and said, "Let's do a little river dance."

I chuckled at his ability to always find humor. While we were still arm-in-arm, I tapped and kicked my feet around like I was dancing. Dave watched me. Then I watched as Dave bent his knees and bounced up and down like he was dancing before we continued down the hall to the bedroom.

"We need to dance to 'From This Moment On,'" I said as I started to half hum and half sing.

"We need more room," he said as we waddled down the hallway while he sang some of the words of our wedding song with me.

As we went through Dave's nightly routine—changing clothes, peeing, organizing stuff on the nightstand—I slowly recited the medication I was leaving for Dave on his nightstand. Before he fell the other night, I used to put his nighttime pain meds in the bathroom. I'd leave a Sharpie and a piece of paper nearby so he could write down the time he took them. In the morning, I'd write the time in the medication journal I've been keeping since we started hospice. This was still in Dave's mind when he mumbled for me to put the medication in the bathroom.

"Dave, you can't walk there by yourself," I said. "Do you want me to put it on my nightstand instead?" He shook his head no.

I'm concerned about his confusion.

16

Sunday, October 22

*D*ave's phone has been living beside the bed, plugged into the charger. His arms have been failing him, and lifting the phone and texting is becoming more difficult. He asked Jessica why his arms are so flaccid. She simply said he is losing strength.

I occasionally check Dave's phone so that I can let him know if he received a text or a phone call. Today, Megan texted her dad, "Good morning, Papa Bear." She often refers to him as Papa Bear in her Facebook posts when updating friends on her father's cancer battle. I know the affectionate term goes back to long before I was a part of their lives.

He responded back to her, "Good morning, Baby Bear."

My heart hurt as I read those words. I let her know it appeared he was going to send another text, but he typed only a couple of letters and never hit send. She appreciated that I told her and asked how my day was going. I told her it was "fine."

I'm not sure how I'm going to keep navigating regular updates to Megan. I want to be truthful, but I know if she has an accurate depiction of Dave's condition it will be impossible for her to stay away. She would want to charge to her dad's side, the same way he charged to the side of his three children any time they were in need. I also know Dave wants her last memory of him to be of a time he was alive.

Several months ago, I asked Dave whether he wants to be buried wearing his wedding band. He hasn't worn it in months. He's lost so much weight he's afraid it will slip off his unusually slender fingers, so he put it in our safe. I hadn't given it much thought. I'd just assumed he should wear it when he's buried. So I asked him. He said yes. Done deal.

Then a week ago, Suzanne Somers died. Dave and I were watching the news and saw an interview with her husband and son. Her husband said he took Suzanne's wedding band and slipped it on a chain that he now wears around his neck. *Hmmm . . . I've never thought of that. I wonder if I should do that,* I thought. When I brought it up to Dave, he told me to do whatever I wanted; he didn't feel strongly one way or the other. I continued to stew over this decision for the next week. One of my flaws is overthinking everything.

I don't know how some decisions become monumental to me, but this one has. It's the proverbial making a mountain out of a molehill. I told Dave a couple of nights ago that I was really stressed over what to do with his wedding band. A familiar look on his face told me he knows how his wife can become obsessed with trivial things. Although realistically, this isn't trivial; this is a one-time decision. Dave told me I needed to buy a good, strong chain for it. This was his way of helping me make the decision.

Last night I pulled Dave's ring out of the safe. I never realized it was white and yellow gold just like my wedding set. I looked through my necklaces to find one I could temporarily use to wear his ring. I settled on my longest yellow-gold chain and slipped it around my neck. As I got ready for bed, I noticed the photograph of Dave and me in a Rolls-Royce, one of Dave's favorite pictures.

It's November 2001, and Dave and I are engaged. Being such a smart guy and a savvy businessman, he qualifies for the big trip again this year. It will be in spring of 2002, one year since we went to Hawaii. This year we are going to Australia, someplace I've always wanted to go and never thought I would.

We decide that we'll probably never find ourselves in the South Pacific again, and the flight is so long from Australia to Los Angeles that we should add a stop. It only makes sense to shorten the trip home if we can, so we decide to spend a few days in Fiji, specifically on Matamanoa Island! As before, the trip is five stars all the way! We spend time in Port Douglas, where I get to snorkel at the Great Barrier Reef in the Coral Sea. The fish and the coral are spectacular!

We also spend time in Sydney shopping and dining. One night we have a five-star experience, as the company hosting the event has outdone itself by arranging a fleet of antique Rolls Royce cars to transport us to dinner. All the couples wait on the red carpet. As the nostalgic cars pull up, we're each handed a flute of champagne and the ladies receive a long-stemmed red rose. We step into the car, momentarily living the lives of the rich and famous as they snap a photo and whisk us away to the Sydney Opera House. We dine like the mega-rich, feeling like royalty, and Dave says, "This is the way in which I ought to be accustomed." That's a Dave-phrase for whenever we're fortunate enough to experience something exceptional.

As I picked up the photo and drank in the memories, I noticed I'd been wearing the watch Dave gave me before the days of fitness watches. I was holding the red rose in my left hand and saw my engagement ring, still solo on my finger. We both looked so happy!

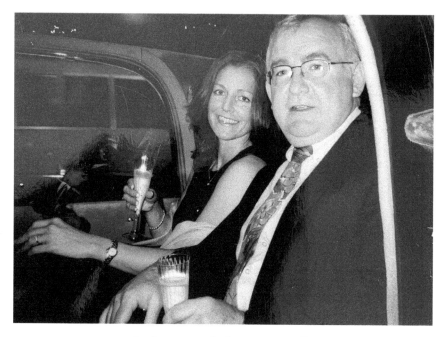

Spring 2002, Sydney, Australia

This morning, when Dave became coherent, I fetched him a drink and some medicine. I sat on the side of the bed, leaning towards him as his wedding band swung free from my neck. "Look what I did with the ring," I said. "I took the beautiful heart pendant off this chain to use for the ring . . . at least temporarily."

"You need a stronger chain," he replied.

"But I don't know if I should get yellow gold or white gold . . . the ring is both," I whined as I rolled the ring in my fingers. Looking up, I realized Dave had drifted back to his other world. My mind wandered back to better days.

> *When Dave and I are in Australia, I don't realize there are traditions being created on our first vacation as a couple. One of them is that Dave will always buy me a gift when we travel. I joke that usually by day three I've had enough togetherness*

and need a day to myself to do my own thing. Eventually I create a routine after we check in to a hotel of immediately scheduling a massage in the spa for mid-week. This becomes the day that Dave usually hunts for my special gift.

On this trip to Sydney, Dave buys me the most exquisite opal I've ever seen. It's in a very unusual setting of white gold on a mid-length chain. I think it's beautiful, but at the time I was wearing mostly yellow gold, so when he gives it to me I start to obsess over whether I should tell him I prefer yellow gold. Generally I don't do well receiving presents, thanks to a rather complicated history with my mother. After two days of stressing over this, I finally tell him. He says we should go to the jewelry store and swap it out for the color gold I want.

We go to the store and explain the scenario. No doubt the jeweler is thinking Dave should snatch the engagement ring off my finger and start "running for the hills," to use one of Dave's regular expressions, before it's too late. I look at both necklaces side by side. They're exactly the same except one is white gold and one is yellow gold. They both have equally stunning stones. Eventually, I come to the realization that Dave was right. The white gold looks better on my skin, and he'd made the right choice in the first place. Now, in spousal jest, I've given him another thing to hold against me for the next twenty years!

Since Dave stays in bed most days, I check on him regularly. Sometimes I climb onto my side of the bed to stroke his face or his arm. Today I told him how much I love him, and he replied, "Know that I'm not in any pain." I smiled and nodded.

Sadie, our sweet pup, has been aware something unusual is going on. My wonderful motherly neighbor and friend has been walking her twice a day. The two have an adorable relationship; I'm not sure who likes whom more.

I leave the front door open, and Joan walks in and calls Sadie. When she returns her when they're done, I occasionally stick my head out of the bedroom and shout, "Thank you, Joanie!" Today after her walk, Sadie came up on the bed with me and Dave. On the rare occasion she joins us, she always lays at the foot. Today she came up near my pillows. I placed Dave's hand on her body. His fingers moved in her blonde hair as she rolled to the side to give him better access.

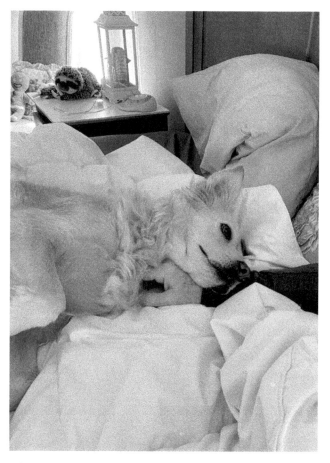

October 22, 2023: Sadie visits Dave; Sloth and Gingerbread
Man linger in the background

*   *   *

My mother came to visit Dave today. My mother and I have an extremely strained relationship. It's more than the usual mother-daughter issues; we have "history." For the last twenty-two years, Dave has been our buffer. I've rarely spent time with my mother unless Dave has been present. He's created an environment where we can exist and keep the tension to a bearable level.

She visited with Dave, spending about ten to fifteen minutes telling him how much she loves him, then said she was going to leave. She didn't leave and continued to carry on a one-sided conversation. It didn't seem to cause Dave any stress, but I wondered how long it would go on. I didn't want to rush her, but I'd told her she had fifteen minutes before she went into the bedroom. She announced again that she was leaving, and Dave suddenly came to life. Not missing a beat, he said with his usual humor, "You're still here." This got a laugh from both of us. Dave and I have always joked that he can say anything to my mother and she never gets mad at him. She knows his teasing is just that: teasing to get a laugh.

After her time with Dave, she came out to the living room with me so we could talk. This visit went okay, but I know it's usually just a matter of time before her visits turn sour and peace is disrupted. Dave's death is tearing her apart, and she has absolutely no one to talk to.

She told me, "No one likes me. But Dave accepts me just the way I am."

She was right on both counts.

Always secretly hoping to ignite a mother-daughter connection, I told her how I'm in the midst of deciding whether to keep Dave's ring around my neck or slip it on his finger when he leaves. She gave me the look. It's the look I've known all my life, the one that says, "I disagree. You're going to regret that. You're making a mistake." There's no mistaking that look; I've seen it too often. I raised my voice slightly and told her to stop it. She's always gotten away with that look because it doesn't accompany words.

She frowned and said, "Dave loves being married, so I think he should wear the ring. Besides, it's not like you're going to wear it for the rest of your life."

As usual, I was disappointed at our interaction.

She spent about six hours at our house today. Eventually, she went back into the bedroom to see Dave, who was completely unresponsive. My mother, extremely upset, cried heavily. I hugged her, something we rarely do, and suggested she sit on the porch in the soothing breezes of the island so she could calm down before she drove herself home. I didn't offer to sit with her. She's often like a vacuum, sucking the life out of everything around her. I need every drop of energy I have to get through what is yet to come.

Jessica came to see Dave in the midst of my mother's visit and was very pleased with the state he's in. He's sleeping almost continuously, doesn't seem to be in any pain, and is actually on very low doses of medication. She said this is ideally how it should be, and she often only sees this when people have said everything they need to say, have no axes to grind, and nothing is keeping them wound up.

Dave slept almost the entire day, and today is the first day he never left the bed. The few moments he was awake since my mother left, he was barely coherent, spending only a few seconds lucid and then skipping off to a more pleasant place in his mind. Today was the first day I realized I can't really talk to him anymore. Well, I can talk to him, but I won't receive a response or acknowledgment. The idea of this is almost paralyzing. Not being able to tell him everything I see and do during the day is one of my greatest fears about losing Dave. The important stuff and the silly stuff, he hears it all.

I don't know how people are supposed to survive this depth of pain. At the moment, I don't even know if I want to. My heart hurts so much, and the fear and dread of the overwhelming grief that is yet to come is incomprehensible. I have cried so much in the last three hours since my mother left that my body is completely drained. I can actually feel pressure at the front of my head between my brows. I think it's from crying.

I finally opened a book I downloaded to my Kindle in the hope it will give me some comfort that "this" isn't all there is ... that our physical life is only a pitstop ... that the body is just a shell ... that there is something more eternal ... that I will see Dave again.

I was so physically drained tonight that I got ready for bed early and climbed in at 7:56 p.m. I spent so many hours today trying to accept that although Dave's body is still here and he's breathing, I won't be able to reach him anymore.

I lay next to him, intending to read more of my book, but all I wanted to do was talk to him. So I closed the book and remembered a monologue I babbled to Dave a few weeks ago:

> *I figure even when you're not here anymore, I'll just keep talking. After all, Dave, for the last twenty-one years, I've spent 90 percent of the time talking, and half that time I'm not really talking to you, I'm just talking. I talk about the dog, the garden, the neighbors, the news. When I do say something that I want you to respond to and you don't answer me, I say, "Dave, are you listening to me?" "Yes, Snooks, I'm listening," you reply.*

Dave had laughed at the time and said I was 100 percent right, that I should keep talking to him when he's no longer here. He knows my talking is a way of reducing anxiety.

He's trying so hard to take care of me. For about two hours, I talked and talked. I stroked his head, arm, and chest the entire time. I was cautious not to drone on about the unbearable pain of losing him. I know he's been worried about me, and I can't add to that worry now. I don't know how much he might be able to comprehend. I certainly talked plenty about how annoyed I am with my mother.

By 10 p.m., I was talked out. Dave had barely moved the entire time. So I did what I've done for the last twenty-one years. I said, "Good night, Bumpy."

"Good night, (mumble)."

My heart skipped! I was shocked that he spoke! I rolled back over to face him. "Bumpy, you know it's your Snookums?" I asked.

"Yes," he said.

"I love you," I told him for the umpteenth time.

"I love you too," he replied.

I have a small plaque on my dresser that says, "Always kiss me good night," and this has been a house rule since the beginning. I said, "Wait, I need my kiss." He rolled his head towards me so I could plant one on his face.

Monday, October 23

J'm still checking Dave's phone periodically. Early this afternoon I saw that Megan sent him another message: "Good afternoon, Papa Bear." The message went unanswered.

Later in the day, I lounged on my side of the bed, to Dave's right, where I was starting to spend more time. Today is the second day Dave hasn't gotten out of bed except to stand to use the pee jug.

While I was lying with him, the doorbell rang. I walked into the hall and looked to the front door, where I saw Patrick. I thought, *Holy shit! What is Patrick doing here?* I headed to the front door to greet him. I was texting with him last night about his dad's latest condition. I asked him when he'd left his house, and he said about twenty minutes after we chatted. He'd driven sixteen hours, through the night, to get here. I was truly elated to see him!

I've listened to Dave tell the story about when baby Patrick was born forty-six years ago. He was very premature, weighing only three pounds, two ounces and ultimately dropping to two pounds, eleven ounces. The nurses in the NICU had to show Dave how to press on little Patrick's chest to restart his heart when he would stop breathing.

Although I didn't know Patrick prior to him being twenty-three years old, he has always appeared to be the most understated and independent of Dave's kids, much like

125

the traits of an only child. Patrick married three years after Dave and I married and is the father of our two oldest grandsons. He's spent the last twenty-two years in law enforcement and quietly continuing his education online. Recently, he became the last of Dave's kids to obtain his doctorate. Dave is insanely proud of all his children and their pursuits of higher education, but Patrick deserves some extra accolades for being able to pursue his degree while simultaneously maintaining his demanding occupation and raising two teenagers with his wife.

As we headed towards the bedroom, I prepared Patrick that Dave may not wake because he's been in and out of consciousness. As we walked in, I loudly said, "Dave, Patrick is here!"

Dave lifted his head off the pillow and looked in the direction of the door. A huge smile crossed his face as he playfully asked, "What the hell are you doing here?"

As he walked around to Dave's side of the bed, Patrick told his father he'd wanted to see him. Dave attempted to sit up, but with his increasing weakness he could lift only a few inches off the pillows as they embraced.

Dave lay back on his pillow and said, "What are you, crazy? Driving all the way from New York?" Dave was absolutely beaming that Patrick was here, and I was ecstatic over the joy on his face.

Within a couple of moments, Dave slipped back into sleep. I took my usual seat on my side of the bed, and Patrick sat on the little stool. We talked about Dave and his condition and discussed hotels for Patrick. Then he left so he could get settled in his room and told me he'd return later.

Megan checked in with a text asking how things were going. I told her, "Long. Weird. Surreal" and let her know her brother showed up today. She immediately said, "I thought dad didn't want us there." I was afraid she was going to jump in the car, and I asked her not to. She assured me she wouldn't.

When Jessica visited today, I explained to her the growing difficulties surrounding Dave's attempts to urinate. I rarely leave the bed because I'm afraid Dave will try to get out of bed on his own. I'm continuing to support as much of his weight as I can while he stands to urinate. When we're sleeping, I hear him stir and ask him if everything is okay. He usually replies, "I have to pee." I race around to his side of the bed as his urgency increases. I help him get his underwear down and hand him the urinal while I wrap my arms under his left arm for support and he grips the jug with his right hand. Dave completes the task and falls back to sleep the second his head lands on the pillow. I dump and rinse the jug and usually find it impossible to go back to sleep for at least an hour or two—it takes some time for the adrenaline jolt to wane. Soon after I fall asleep, Dave has to urinate again.

Same process, again and again.

The entire experience is exhausting for him. Honestly, the entire experience is exhausting for me too. And every time we do this, I notice he's able to support less of his weight. Each time it takes longer and longer for Dave to feel he has voided his bladder sufficiently, but each time there's less and less volume in the jug and the color indicates his dehydration is continuing. His urgency to pee increases, as does his panic that he won't get to the jug in time.

Jessica suggested a catheter. Dave said no. He doesn't want a catheter. I feel it's in his, and certainly in my, best interest, but I want to respect his wishes. Instead, she ordered us some "adult briefs," also known as diapers, as well as some "pee pads" I can put on the bed in case of accidents.

I asked her to look at the pressure sore developing on Dave's tush. He has a scratch on his buttock, most likely from the urgent grasping to get his underwear down quickly. Dave has fingernail clippers in every corner of the house and used to keep his fingernails very short. Now they are far longer.

Jessica suggested I keep a barrier cream on any pressure sores and try to rotate Dave's position more frequently.

I've added these tasks to the daily regimen.

Tuesday, October 24

"Good morning, Papa Bear" appeared on Dave's phone again this morning. I didn't even see it for a while because Dave's care has become all-consuming.

Since Patrick's arrival, he has been tasked with updating Megan on their father's condition. He's gentler with his words. I have a reputation for not sugarcoating anything, and that direct approach would not be beneficial now.

Patrick and I spend the entire day talking, sitting with Dave while he sleeps. I am relieved someone is here during the day so I can leave the bed for a moment to go to the bathroom or get a cup of coffee.

Today I decided to switch Dave to adult diapers. I don't even know how to tell Dave I'm putting a diaper on him. I guess I could call them adult briefs, as Jessica suggested, to prevent embarrassment for Dave. At this point, I don't even know if he would be embarrassed. I'm just trying to do everything right.

These adult briefs are nearly impossible for Dave to remove. They're even difficult for me to remove because the edge of the tab is hard to find. They're clearly not designed for someone who wants to be self-sufficient. These are designed for someone who's bed-bound, possibly in a coma, and has no control over their bowels or bladder. With my truck-driver language, I frequently cuss that these must have been designed by a fucking sadist as I fumble for the tabs, trying to help Dave with the pee process every few hours.

Dave continues to lean against the bed for support when he has to pee. Patrick is assisting me in holding Dave's right side as I continue to support his weight on his left side, but when

I'm alone at night I wrap my arms around his waist; it's the only way I can hold him. He often has to pee at about 2 a.m. I fall back to sleep around 4 a.m. and then get maybe two hours of sleep until he has to go again. I'm not sure how I'm functioning on so little sleep.

Wednesday, October 25

At 8 this morning, I texted Margaret: "I think I need you to come down. I'm wrestling with decisions that are good for him versus what he wants. And I think I just need your support to help me through this." The decision I was referring to is the catheter. I hit the send button.

A short time later, her response came through that she would let me know her travel arrangements as soon as she had them. I knew there would be no delay in her response. Margaret, and her partner Claire, made it very clear they would be available to me at any time, for whatever I needed, for however long I needed it. Even though I've visualized that I'll be the only person with Dave at the end of his life, all along I've known Margaret would be my go-to person, if necessary. Even Dave mentioned to me one day that if things get tough to call his sister for help. I don't ask for help easily, but I need help, both for Dave and for myself. I can't hold him up alone anymore, especially for the increasing amount of time it's been taking for him to pee in the middle of the night.

Margaret didn't bat an eye. She told me she could come at midnight tonight or 1 p.m. tomorrow. I wrestled with the decision. I know Dave would not want me to inconvenience his sister by asking her to arrive at midnight. I also know he would not want me to handle this alone when I'm struggling. I bounced the idea off Patrick, the person I now think out loud to.

I told Margaret that midnight would be great. She said she could take a car service from the airport and that I should leave the front door unlocked. I was incredibly relieved to hear she was coming. I know the emotional support she can provide is immense.

After I finished messaging with her, I whispered to Dave, "I called Margaret. She's coming." Dave nodded his head in approval.

I tried to freshen up Dave by wiping his face with a warm washcloth, brushing his hair, and changing him into his BEAST T-shirt. I don't know if it actually made him feel any better, I know it used to, but I'm afraid it might be benefiting only me now. It was Dr. Thorn who first called Dave a beast, after his complete rhinectomy. Dave was out of the hospital in record time, and during one of our follow-up visits, Dr. Thorn said, "You're a beast." Dave loved that! That's when I bought him the blue T-shirt with the white letters BEAST. All of us close to Dave have been calling him a beast ever since.

Since Patrick has been here, we've spent a tremendous amount of time talking. He spends about twelve hours a day with me. I sit on my side of the bed with my back against the headboard, and Patrick sits in the chair beside Dave. I've removed the little stool and replaced it with a dining room chair for Patrick to sit on. The not-overly-comfortable stool for visitors was intentional so people would keep their visits short. But poor Patrick showed up here with a crutch in hand because he's having some difficulty with his back and his legs.

The first couple of times Dave had to pee while his son was here, Patrick left the room to allow his dad some privacy. Now Patrick stays to help me. I've switched Dave back to underwear since the damned diapers were so hard to open. I'm not worried about Dave having an accident; I'll deal with it if it happens. Although his body is shrinking by the day, his weight seems significant to both of us.

Dave's attempts to urinate have become somewhat urgent and panicked. The second he reaches to lift the blankets from his body, I ask him if he has to pee. He nods, then moves robotically as his primal need continues. Patrick and I get into position as I hand the jug to Dave. It seems to be taking several minutes, but it's probably no more than two. Dave stands with only his toes on the floor; all his ligaments and tendons bulge in his once-muscular calves as he uses every ounce of strength to stand.

He continues to have significant bladder pressure but has trouble getting the urine out. He often thrusts his hips in an attempt to void, making it even more difficult to hold him. I also try to assist in holding the jug because I'm afraid Dave will drop it. At times the urine splashes or starts early and dribbles to the carpet. Dave mumbles that I'll have to have the carpets cleaned; I tell him not to worry about it and spray some vinegar to neutralize any odor. Eventually I'll get the carpet cleaned, but for now I'm using one of the pee pads supplied by hospice to cover the floor. I've also put one under the fitted sheet in our bed in case Dave eventually voids in his sleep. The experience has become exhausting, not only for Dave but for Patrick and me.

Dave's arms are becoming like spaghetti; he has so little control over them. He raises an arm to touch his face, which he does often, and it just collapses. I begin to gently support his elbow at the height needed, as he can still control his hands and fingers.

I have now moved an even more comfortable chair next to the bed for Patrick. It's the pink chair from the living room, the one Dave used to sit in when accepting his visitors. Dave is never left alone . . . not for a minute.

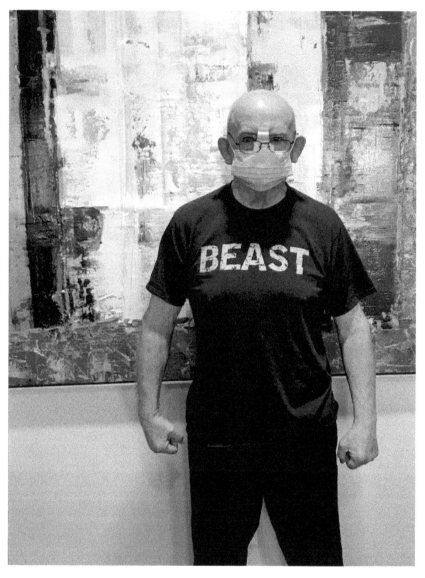

July 2021: Dave proudly wears his BEAST T-shirt

18

Thursday, October 26

*A*round 12:30 a.m., I woke to hear Sadie barking. Margaret was coming through the front door I'd left unlocked for her. I got out of bed realizing I was actually in the middle of a good sleep that had lasted more than three hours. I greeted her and told her the gist of what's been going on. I returned to bed quickly, hoping to jump back into sleep mode. Margaret settled herself in our guest room down the hall.

A couple of hours later, I felt Dave move. It was the usual drill: I asked him if he had to pee, his responses were much less verbal, but nevertheless I understood the answer was yes.

"Margaret!" I called as I ran to Dave's side of the bed. "Margaret!" I shouted again.

Margaret wears a CPAP, and I worry that this arrangement is not going to work. How will she be able to help me in the middle of the night if she can't hear me? I don't want to shout her name again because I assume my shouting voice will become increasingly upsetting to Dave.

Dave is so frail he cannot even sit up by himself, but he moves on autopilot, flipping back the covers with urgency as I grasp his arms and help move his feet to the floor. He sits on the edge of the bed for a moment, playing a balancing act. Apparently the urge to pee is not as severe as it usually is. I tell him I'll be right back.

I run down the hall, flipping on the light as I go. I get to Margaret's open door and slam the palm of my hand on the door twice while bellowing, "Get up!"

Margaret rips off her CPAP mask and follows me back to Dave's bedside. As I'm attempting to lift his left arm to raise him to his feet, she follows my lead by securing his right, and in her normal, cheerful way she sings, "Hellooo Bruddah!" She continues to look over Dave's shoulder as I help him lower his underwear and hand him the jug. He wants to hold the jug himself, but he has such tremors over his body that the jug keeps splashing and nearly slipping out of his hands. I'm glad I'd placed the pee pad beneath where we're standing.

Dave holds the jug as I support it from the bottom. I wish he could sit on the edge of the bed while he urinates, but he's still determined to stand. I imagine the prostate of a seventy-year-old man might not be cooperative with sitting and urinating.

Margaret and I firmly hold Dave in place while he continues to tremor and he thrusts his hips. He never feels like he has emptied his bladder. When some time has passed and there's no more liquid dripping into the jug, I gently and quietly say, "Bumps, I think you're done now."

He says no. Just no.

We continue to hold him in place, both of us straining under the weight of his helpless body. He's reluctant to let me peel his fingers off the jug, but eventually he does so. It's almost as if his right hand has cramped around the handle.

We lower his body to sit on the side of the bed. I have no idea what's going through his head. He points to the pink chair in front of him.

"Bumpy, you want to sit on the pink chair?" I ask.

He nods.

The pee pad beneath our feet is bunching up, making it difficult to raise Dave and move him the 180 degrees he needs to turn to sit in the chair. I tell Margaret I believe I'd be more successful doing this alone.

"Bumpy, I'm going to wrap my arms around your waist and turn you," I say.

He's afraid of falling and tries to help. I continue to assure him I will not drop him.

"Trust me, Bumps, I will not drop you," I confidently whisper.

I can almost pick him up while holding him in this position. He is so frail I am nearly afraid I will break his bones. I turn him so his back is towards the pink chair. "Bumps, I'm going to lower you . . . bend your knees . . . I won't drop you . . . I promise you," I assure him.

Margaret hovers in the tiny space where Dave now spends his days and nights—between the bed and the pink chair. Dave lowers to the chair and seems relieved to be sitting. I wonder how much of his disorientation is from the drugs and how much is due to this period of transitioning.

This is the first time someone other than me is able to see what transpires at night in our bedroom. I am sure Margaret sees why I need her here. She sits on the bed and chats with her brother. Dave doesn't speak. Other than saying when he has to pee or pointing to the chair or the bed, all we hear from Dave is an occasional murmur.

At 4 a.m., Dave tells me he wants a slushie. I'm astounded! I rush to the kitchen, leaving Dave in Margaret's care. I whip together the pineapple—or maybe it was mango—Italian ice and pineapple-orange juice in the blender.

When I come back, I feed the slushie to Dave. He is unable to hold anything of any weight in his hands. The weakness, which was only in his upper arms, is now affecting his lower arms as well as his hands and fingers. Even when he attempts to grab a tissue, his arms collapse.

I hand him the tissue, tuck it in his fingers, and support his elbow in a position so he can blot whatever he feels needs blotting. He constantly attempts to wipe his upper lip. I assume this is from the habitual preoccupation over the last two years that his nose hole is leaking blood or mucus. Often, the tissue falls from his fingers to the floor, and I can see on his face he recognizes that he's unable to hold a tissue. I'm sure he's internally frustrated, but he does an amazing job at not holding onto that frustration or taking it out on us. He just smirks and sighs.

He takes only a few swallows of the slushie. I think back to the blue pamphlet from hospice: *The body knows it does not need food any longer.* This is the last solid food Dave will ever take in. His body has reached a state of emaciation. His ribs and hips protrude severely. His legs and arms are like spaghetti and of no use to him except to robotically grab the pee jug. I'm not sure how he can reach for the jug when he can't even hold a tissue.

Eventually Dave points to the bed and mumbles he wants to go back to bed. I reverse the belly hold I did before. It's slightly more difficult to lift him, as the chair is lower than the bed. I have a chronic bad back and know the chances are great that one of these times I'm going to do some considerable damage to my back. My only concern is how I'll be able to move Dave if that happens.

I turn Dave the 180 degrees, promising him the whole time I will not drop him, and seat him on the bed. It's now close to 5:30 a.m., and Margaret and I are exhausted. We've been having difficulty getting Dave into a sleeping position. Somehow, all three of us roll onto the bed like Weebles. Overtired and overstressed, Margaret and I laugh. As we roll, my biggest concern is Dave falling back on the bed with his feet on the floor, which would hurt his back. I want to do everything right.

We finally manage to spin him ninety degrees, but he's far too close to the foot of the bed. We need to slide him up at least a foot towards the headboard. I don't know how someone so tiny can weigh so much. I employ my brain to work smarter, not harder, as I visualize every senior dog I've had to move that weighed over seventy-five pounds. I suggest we roll a towel under Dave and use that to lift his hips into position. I straddle over Dave like a sumo wrestler, one end of the towel wrapped around each hand, lifting with my legs and not my back while Margaret gets in position to prop pillows. Eventually I'm satisfied with Dave's sleeping position. I slip another pillow under his calves to relieve the pressure on his heels. I coat his lips with olive oil, something I do at least a dozen times a day to keep his lips from drying out, then Margaret and I return to our beds.

I wonder if she realized it was going to be this bad.

That it was going to be this hard.

Things are worsening exponentially.

We get a couple of hours of sleep before Patrick comes over. The three of us surround Dave constantly. Patrick most often sits in the pink chair, which he has scooted close enough to the bed that he can stroke his dad's arm or hold his hand. At times, I look over at Patrick, his forehead on the bed, always touching his father. I know this experience will change him forever, the way it has changed me.

Megan continues to message Patrick to request updates. Mere moments after Patrick's response, Margaret's phone will ping. Megan has an insatiable need for information—no different than I would be—but the information that is disseminated outside this room is very strategic and agreed upon by all before the written word is sent out. There is no need for anyone to suffer while sitting at home knowing how unbearable being witness to Dave's death actually is.

We continue to talk to Dave as if he can hear us. Maybe he can . . . maybe he can't. But we all love him so dearly and respect him so much, we want to make him a part of our conversations.

For just a few moments, Margaret and I find ourselves sitting on the living room sofa. Patrick is keeping a watchful eye on his father. I tell Margaret that I stopped writing in my journal. I've shared the very early stages with Claire, telling her I may actually see if I can get this published. "People need to know about this kind of love," I told her. "People need to know about this kind of pain. And I hope I can say someday that people need to know they can survive this kind of pain."

Margaret asks me why I stopped writing.

"How can I preserve Dave's dignity? He would be mortified if people knew he pooped in his pants during the night. Nobody told me that was going to happen. Nobody told me how hard this would be. Every person I've ever heard about who died in hospice, every announcement on the news about a celebrity death, is described with the words, 'He died peacefully surrounded by his family.' That's such bullshit!" I rant. "Every part of this is hard. Hard for Dave, hard for me. What about the constant urinating? And the thrusting hips? Nobody ever tells you that's going to happen. The tremors? What about that? Never heard about that. The way his right foot got all weird like he was stepping over a log. What about that? I read that blue pamphlet front to back more than once and none of that is in there!"

Margaret replies, "Well, maybe somebody needs to tell them."

"What about Dave's dignity?" I plea. "I don't want to do anything that would embarrass him."

"Do you think any less of Dave after seeing all this firsthand?"

"No! I think he's the bravest, most loving man I've ever known. He's been so incredibly strong and patient with all of us."

"Then isn't that what other people will see too? Maybe people need to know. Maybe someone needs to tell the story of what can happen when someone is dying."

Margaret's words roll around in my head over the next few hours.

In the afternoon, I ask out loud if anyone notices the swelling on the left side of Dave's face . . . the "non-cancer" side. His head has been slightly turned to the left, and I'm hoping it's just an illusion, but it seems apparent there is swelling. It stems from below his ear and runs all the way up to his temple. Since Thursdays are one of Jessica's days off, I text her and send her pictures. She calls and suggests it may be lymph node swelling and suggests I try alternating hot and cold compresses, which might bring down the swelling. She will be by first thing Friday morning.

My journal of medication is becoming incredibly necessary. Dave still has a 50-mcg fentanyl patch on, which I change every forty-eight hours. He also takes 30 mg of morphine every four hours, 4 mg of dexamethasone in the morning, and 0.5 mg of lorazepam every six hours. I have alarms set throughout the day and night. I'm crushing pills, mixing them with the morphine, and drawing it all up in a plastic syringe in order to get Dave's medicine safely into his mouth. He spends so little time awake.

This afternoon I moved Dave to the pink chair, hoping we may see a reduction of the swelling in his face if he's sitting upright. I never would have moved him if he hadn't been agreeable, but he was. I don't remember who suggested Dave might like to listen to music, but I decided to give it a try. I pulled out my phone and scrolled down to Simon and Garfunkel.

"The Sound of Silence" plays. Dave immediately reacts with a smile. He tilts his head and nods, his face softens; he hears the music. His eyes that were half closed widen for just a moment. With his arms resting on the pink chair, he raises a forearm and points a finger. I believe he is moving to the music as a conductor of an orchestra; Margaret thinks he is gesturing to greet the darkness of his other world. Either way, I'm glad to have been able to bridge our worlds, if just for a moment.

Friday, October 27

*T*here has been a little brass-colored bell on Dave's nightstand for weeks. It used to live in our curio, which is filled with other sentimental items. Dave's mother used to give this bell to her kids when they were sick. My mother did the same thing with me so I could ring it from bed when I needed something. I pulled it out of the curio and gave it to Dave when he was mobile yet needed my help and his failing voice wouldn't reach me if I were in another room.

Margaret and I decided I should move the bell to my nightstand, ringing it in the middle of the night when I needed her to help me with Dave. Maybe the difference in tone will help her wake out of a deep sleep. She can't understand how the sound of a cat ready to cough up a furball will vault her out of bed and across the room, and yet she has difficulty hearing me call at night.

Sometime in the early morning hours, Dave signals it's time for the urgent pee ritual. I shout out to Margaret and ring the little golden bell. I don't hear her coming down the hall. Damn!

I shout a second time.

I still don't hear Margaret.

I've gone back to putting the adult briefs on Dave because it has become necessary, and I'm urgently attempting to pull these damned tabs off this sadistic diaper he's trapped in. I desperately claw at the tape. *Who designed these things?!*

I position Dave on the edge of the bed, jug in my hand. I don't know how to wake Margaret, but I know I need her help if Dave is going to stand.

Think, Patty. Damn it, think!

I look for what I can throw. I grab the jar of ointment I've been using for Dave's pressure sores and throw it through the doorway, hoping it will hit the hall wall, fall onto the floor, and roll over to Margaret's room. My aim is spot-on. I wonder if I'll find a hole in the sheetrock in the morning.

I still don't hear Margaret. I assume the rolling jar woke her and she's lying there waiting for another sound, not sure what woke her. I call her name one more time, and she comes running in to assist.

Dave continues to be incredibly patient with us. We grab, we fuss, we do the best we can. He never gets angry. I don't know how he has become so tolerant. In truth, he was never this tolerant when he was healthy. Cancer has changed both of us so much. I never imagined we would have infinite patience with one another under such extreme circumstances. Our love for each other has continued to grow throughout this journey. I've been unable to find an accurate word that depicts what we have between us—something more than love—so I've settled on describing it as Dave is now part of my soul.

Hours later, Pastor Bobby pops in unexpectedly. We continue to address Dave in our conversations as if he is lucid. After I announce, "Dave, Bobby is here," we are all so surprised and our eyes widen as Dave opens his eyes and turns his head to the bedroom door. He manages a rumbly sounding, "Hey Bob."

Bobby stays for about five minutes, "loving up on" Dave and me. We pray before he leaves. I'm afraid Bobby will be the last visitor Dave ever sees.

We're anxious for Jessica's arrival. I'm concerned about crackles in Dave's breathing. After he exhales, it sounds almost like a paper bag crinkling. With Dave's history of pneumonia, we fear that's what this is. Since one of the requirements for Margaret to obtain her thanatology certification has involved her being present during the passing of others, I ask her if this is the death rattle I've heard so much about. She says it's not.

Dave's face is still swollen. Maybe it has dissipated ever so slightly. Maybe that's wishful thinking.

Jessica arrives and we share our concerns with her. She examines Dave and says his heart is strong and his lungs are clear, something every nurse who has taken his vitals has said. I'm still amazed that his heart is so strong. Before cancer, Dave was relatively healthy. He was a self-described "middle-aged, fat White guy" and took meds associated with that description. High blood pressure and high cholesterol have been an issue for the last couple of decades, the usual conditions for a man who has spent more time behind a desk than on a treadmill and more time eating what tasted good, not necessarily what was healthy. I've generally cooked healthy food for our meals, but Dave usually follows it up with a large coffee mug packed with vanilla ice cream. He hasn't had an indulgence like that for years. Not since cancer. Cancer stole that pleasure from him.

We decide to double Dave's fentanyl patch to 100 mcg. I will change it every seventy-two hours. We also add on hyoscyamine, one of the five drugs from the comfort pack, every twelve hours to keep the mucus from thickening. He's already so dry from the radiation he had nearly three years ago that we don't want to dry him out too much.

We again address the idea of a catheter. I desperately want to honor Dave's wishes, but the mental and physical stress and strain of attempting to get out of bed is so demanding for him—for all of us. We cannot comprehend how he musters the energy to do it. He's definitely on autopilot when he feels the urge to urinate. Not to mention, it's taking three of us to hold Dave for the five-plus minutes it takes him to feel he has emptied his bladder. And he used to pee over a half cup; now it's just a few tablespoons. Jessica believes that since he's unable to empty his bladder completely, that urge comes more frequently. I decide it's in his best interest to insert the catheter. I ask Margaret and Patrick if they agree. They do.

Dave, Jessica, and I are alone in the bedroom when she inserts the catheter. This is the first expression of pain I have seen on Dave's face in days. Jessica tells me she's having some difficulty getting around his prostate. I try to soothe Dave with whispers of comfort while she assures me he will not remember the discomfort.

The last time Dave had a catheter was three years ago after his first surgery at the university hospital. I remember being so upset that the "teaching nurse" was having difficulty at the expense of Dave. I am amazed at how much I have learned about cancer since then. How much I have learned about life. How much I have learned about love.

As soon as the catheter is inserted, urine runs into the bag. Dave is peacefully unaware. I know I made the right choice. We close his adult briefs, and Jessica provides me instructions on emptying the urine bag if necessary. I've read that eventually, his urine will turn a dark tea color and thicken like honey. Jessica confirms this. For now, it's still dark yellow and liquid.

Dave has been drinking no more than four ounces a day for the last few days, and he hasn't taken in any fluids today. I keep thinking back to that blue pamphlet: *The body knows it no longer needs liquid.* I ask where all the urine is coming from. Jessica says since the body is 90 percent water, it's now purging liquid from his cells. I'm aware that this means his organs are rapidly deteriorating.

Patrick and Margaret step into the bedroom while I walk Jessica to the door and try to get a better feel for how much time we have left. I'm not sure what the difference would be if it were one day, one week, or one month, but I've always had the need to know what's ahead of me. She says, "I fully expect to see both of you on Monday."

Colonel Tom is coming back from Hawaii very late tonight. Yesterday, I texted him and told him we're wondering whether Dave is holding on for his return. Tom has been gone for ten days and would feel horrible if Dave died before he had a chance to say goodbye. If it were up to Dave, he would never let Tom live with that guilt. We plan for Tom to come to the house on Saturday morning.

This afternoon Dave wakes and wants to pee. He goes into autopilot, attempting to flip the covers back and get out of bed by himself. Before he can move, I grab his arms, fearful he will try to rip out the catheter. I sit on the bed in my usual spot, gently restraining both of Dave's arms. He is frail and fragile, yet he is still strong.

He urgently cries out, "I gotta pee, I gotta pee!"

I quietly assure him, "It's okay Bumps. You have a catheter. You don't have to go anywhere."

He continues, "I gotta pee, I gotta pee!"

"It's okay Bumpy . . . you have a catheter . . . the pee will go right in the bag," I quietly whisper to him so as not to agitate him more.

The love . . . the trust . . . the bond we have calms Dave and he acquiesces. He seems content and relaxes his body. He's asleep within seconds.

I'm happy we have the catheter but devastated at the turmoil that seems to be going on inside him. *Is Dave still here? Can he hear us? Is he hanging on for Tom? Does he feel any pain?* These thoughts circle through my head continuously. My OCD is relentless.

Jessica tells me the signs to look for that would indicate whether Dave is experiencing breakthrough pain. If this happens, I should give him more morphine.

I make sure Dave appears comfortable at all times. I spend more and more time whispering in his ear . . . telling him how much I love him . . . whispering, "Don't forget the blue butterfly."

Over these cancer-filled years, I have shared my fears with Dave about there being nothing after this life . . . about it just being "over-over," as I call it. Dave knew this about me, and it's been something we've discussed over the years. I've reminded him many times that he needs to let me know he's okay . . . to let me know there is more than just this existence.

During our marriage, Dave has had a habit of opening a kitchen cabinet, taking what he needs, then leaving the cabinet door open as he exits the room. This used to drive me crazy! I used to say, "One of these days you're going to bang your head so hard on that open door you'll remember to close it from then on." We've decided that this will be the sign. After he dies, if he really becomes a spirit watching over me, if there's any way that's possible, he will open a cabinet door and leave it open. He has reminded me of this over the last couple of years when he's seen me worry. He'll say, "Just look for the open cabinet." That usually pulls a smile out of me.

Since my experience meeting Chris-on-the-beach, the blue butterfly has come to symbolize that there is something else out there. God? The universe? Other souls that have passed on and are trying to help us mere mortals? Several times a day since Dave has become bedridden, I whisper, "Don't forget the blue butterfly."

Dave has been sleeping peacefully for about forty minutes. At about 4 p.m., I leave the bed for the kitchen. I have never sat so long in my entire life, and my body is feeling the effects of the lack of movement. I stretch my legs and wander around looking in the fridge and on the counter for food that's appealing. No more than five minutes later, I hear Margaret and Patrick's voices yell, "Patty!"

I run into the bedroom, then slide into my position on the bed like a ball player sliding into home base. Dave is stirring. As he wakes, he urgently says, "I gotta pee, I gotta pee!"

This time he is more agitated. This time he has more strength. I don't want to hurt him by wrestling him, and I don't want to pin his arms, but we need to protect him from yanking out the catheter. I try saying all the soothing words that worked less than an hour ago. It's not working.

"Margaret, get my phone and call Jessica," I call out.

Margaret puts the phone on speaker and places it near me on the bed. I can feel the panic coming through Dave. He's desperately trying to sit up. He twists and turns. His adrenaline gives him more strength than he should have.

"Patrick, keep holding his left arm," I say. It's dangerously near the catheter. I continue to hold his right arm while leaning across his legs, trying to keep him from swinging them out of bed. I know what Jessica is going to say.

I remember the day Myra went over the emergency pack of comfort drugs we were supposed to have on hand. When she mentioned haloperidol for agitation, my eyes had teared at the thought of what was ahead for Dave and me.

Jessica says to give Dave 1.0 mg of haloperidol. Margaret drops a tablet into his mouth and tries to get it under his tongue. His agitation continues.

"I gotta pee, I gotta pee!" he continues to cry out.

This is heartbreaking for all of us. Dave doesn't understand what is happening. I pray the haloperidol works fast. It seems to take an eternity, but after a half hour or so Dave succumbs. His muscles relax. He starts to lie back in bed. I hold both his arms, more gently now, assuring him he can relax everything.

"Bumpy, don't worry. You won't pee the bed," I tell him.

With the wide eyes of a four-year-old child, and in a voice that nearly matches, he asks, "Are you sure?"

"Yes, Dave. Just relax. Relax everything," I softly say.

He returns with, "Are you sure I won't pee in the bed?"

He is darling and sweet and so very vulnerable. My heart is breaking into a million pieces as I see the man I love, the man who has spent his life helping everyone he knows, being so vulnerable. I'm afraid that this is the last conversation I will have with my sweet Dave.

Dave drifts into sleep as the haloperidol does its job. Pulling out the medication journal, I make notes to dose him with it every six hours and increase the lorazepam to every four.

I don't want to leave Dave's side. Margaret and Patrick often bring me coffee and food, regularly urging me to eat. I've showered maybe twice in the last week. I get an average of four, maybe five hours of sleep a night. Although I'm ready to collapse by 8 p.m., Dave needs morphine and lorazepam at 9 p.m. and haloperidol at 10 p.m. Before bed, I go to the kitchen just long enough to crush pills and measure out meds. I set everything on my nightstand with sticky notes, afraid I'll be disoriented when my alarm goes off. My alarm is set for 1 a.m. and 5 a.m. I hope that I'm able to get back to sleep between those times.

I am fairly certain, now that Dave has started the haloperidol, he will never speak to me again. I cope with that thought by knowing I will never see pain, fear, or panic in his eyes again.

The bedroom has become somewhat of an inner sanctum. It feels sacred. It's where I live nearly twenty-four hours a day, and Margaret and Patrick, probably eighteen. The connection between the three of us is deepening. We're close to being able to communicate without words. This has been a life-changing experience for all.

Gradually over the last few days, a sort of unspoken seating hierarchy has developed in the bedroom. My seat is seat

number one, next to Dave on the bed. It's the seat of prominence because it's closest to him and belongs to his wife. It's
the seat that allows me to have several parts of my body touching his, a seat where I can whisper in his ear the things I need
him to hear. The second seat is the pink chair next to the bed.
Patrick occupies this seat most of the time. From there, he can
stroke Dave's arm or touch his upper body. Since poor Patrick
arrived here with a crutch under his arm, he needs a chair of
substance.

The dining chair, which we've moved to the foot of the
bed, has become the third seat. By default, Margaret often
occupies this seat, sometimes slipping her hands under the
sheet to hold Dave's feet. When I leave my seat for only a few
moments, Margaret seamlessly glides into position one so she
can gently stroke Dave's arm or hold a cool compress to his
forehead. When I return, she pops up like toast from a toaster
to let me resume my position. At times, when I return with
food in hand, I often take the seat at the foot of the bed, silently
nodding to her to stay where she is as I prop my feet next to
Dave's and observe the room from a different view. When the
food is gone, there's no need for me to nudge Margaret out of
my seat. She's always ready to quietly offer it back and resume
her foothold.

The same process takes place when Patrick vacates the
pink chair. Margaret will move up a notch into seat number
two, only until his return. As Dave's sister, Margaret is certainly no less important to Dave than Patrick and me. However, she has an extraordinary sensitivity to appreciating and
valuing the relationships of wife and son.

This has become how we've been maneuvering for days.
We're like volleyball players sliding into position when it's
time to rotate. I climb into bed, then secure Dave's arms over
the blanket so that in the event he wakes up he won't be able
to grab at his catheter. It's chilly, so I put a comforter over

both of us. I snuggle up as close as I can, always careful not to hurt his fragile body. I whisper how much I love him and how happy I am that I married him. I stop myself from saying anything about not knowing how I'll continue a happy life without him. Although I don't know how I will, I'm afraid if he can hear me at all, that will make him sad. I don't want him to be sad.

Lately, Dave's breathing has become so loud that I've been using earplugs at night. I don't know whether it's congestion, sleep apnea, or something else. I can still hear his breath, but the plugs drown out the noise enough that I can get some sleep. If he so much as twitches, I wake up. I basically sleep with one eye open.

Dave's breathing changes during the night enough to wake me up. I can see his silhouette thanks to the low-watt lamp I placed on his nightstand weeks ago. I reach to touch him. He feels like he's burning up. But his T-shirt isn't soaked like it usually is when he gets night sweats. I slip my hand under his arms and neck. He feels like he's on fire. His head is warm but not burning. I pull the comforter off him and cover him with a bright-blue sheet.

I pull out the pulse oximeter we've had in the house for weeks but have rarely used; it now sits on my nightstand. Patrick bought it days ago when he bought a rubber donut to soften the seat on the pink chair for Dave. Dave's oxygen level is still in the 80s. I grab the nasal cannula and slip it between Dave's lips. I trot out to the living room, past Margaret's room to where the oxygen concentrator sits, and flip it on. The machine beeps loudly when first turned on, waking Margaret. As I return past her room, I stick my head in and say, "I'm going to give him some oxygen."

I think of a text that Tracey sent me earlier this evening after she stopped by the house to drop something off and saw the oxygen. I hadn't even come out to greet her; Margaret and Patrick were addressing anyone who stopped by. She told me that when she was caring for her dad in his last days, no one told her to stop using oxygen when his pulse ox dropped below seventy. She said she believed the oxygen prevented him from passing four days sooner than he would have.

I'm worried that I will prolong Dave's life unnecessarily. When we enlisted the help of hospice, I told Dave, "I will support you and every breath you take as long as you want to be here, but the minute you decide you're done . . . that's it."

I want to do everything right.

20

Saturday, October 28

I text Molly and tell her our nurse is off for the weekend. I want to know how low a person's oxygen level can go before deciding to stop administering oxygen.

At least two years ago, I was at the gym and decided to take a yoga class, Molly was the instructor. She's of average height and build and has long, blonde curls. She also has a wild expression of herself emblazoned on her body with tattoos, as well as a calming energy that can't be missed. I've been taking her classes weekly, as they're offered only on Saturday mornings. The class is good, but the feeling of life I get from Molly's class is better than good—it's energizing and restores the soul. I even bring Megan to the class when she's visiting. She agrees that this class is special.

After speaking with Molly, I eventually learn she's a hospice nurse. Wow! My mind immediately wonders if our meeting is not a chance encounter. Dave has already been diagnosed with cancer, and I wonder whether it's possible Molly and I met at the gym so that we could bond before her real purpose to me becomes evident: to support me when my husband dies and to usher him during his passing.

Months pass, and Molly's hours change to working weekends, not weekdays. She's a visiting hospice nurse, and it occurs to me that our meeting at yoga may be insignificant. Then Molly is diagnosed with a particularly nasty cancer. Being that I'm living on the cancer train, I'm able to be supportive in ways I wouldn't have been years ago. Now I wonder if our meeting was intentional so that I'd be able to comfort her and not the other way around.

Once Dave and I enlist the help of hospice, I occasionally reach out to Molly with questions. It's easier to talk to her about things I wouldn't speak to the four different nurses we've had in a month's time. Molly replies with detailed, informative, carefully worded responses. She also checks in on me often via text, sending big red heart emojis and reminding me I am loved. I live just over the county line she serves in, so I realize she will never be my hospice nurse, but her support has been crucial.

Molly tells me that oxygen is gauged by comfort. If Dave is breathing comfortably without the oxygen, she gives the option to remove it. If his breathing gets labored after removing it, we can put it back on.

"Who is your on-call nurse?" she asks.

I tell her I really don't want to see a new nurse; we've already had four. Molly tells me she's working this weekend and asks if I'd like her to visit. I would love for her to visit.

When Molly gets to the house, I meet her at the door. She's wearing her long-sleeved scrubs, so her tattoos aren't visible. Her long, wild hair is spun in a tight little bun, and she's wearing wire-rimmed glasses. Her physical transformation from yoga instructor to hospice nurse is obvious, but the comforting look on her face is the same.

The minute I see her I start to cry. She holds me and comforts me. When we hug, she places her hand behind my head and holds me close, the way a mother would with her child. I walk her to the bedroom. She has an energy and presence that relaxes everyone the minute she walks in. I introduce her to Margaret and Patrick, and of course, I introduce her to Dave.

"Dave, honey," I say, "remember Molly, the yoga instructor I told you about who's also a hospice nurse? She's here."

Molly addresses Dave as if he were sitting there with eyes wide open. "Dave, it's such a pleasure to meet you. I've heard so much about you," she warmly says.

I share my concerns about Dave's breathing and the heat coming off his body. She examines him, always prefacing her actions with words: "Dave, I am going to pick up your right arm . . . Dave, I am going to touch your left leg." Her calming demeanor and gentle touch is like a warm blanket on a cold night. The tension in the room has been at an all-time high, yet she is able to diffuse it with her presence.

Molly is confident that Dave is not in pain and that his breathing is not labored. I explain my fear that since Dave's breathing sounds different, I'm afraid he can't get enough air. She asks if I notice a difference when I put the oxygen on him. No, there is no change in his breathing; only the pulse oximeter increases. She says that the oxygen is probably not helping him, but he also doesn't seem to be struggling. She continues to provide a calming presence. Her voice is soothing. She treats Dave as if he were her dad, continuing to care for him gently.

"Dave, I'm going to swab out your mouth a bit," she tells him. "You'll feel some cool water and a small sponge." She shows me how to wipe out his mouth with the sponge, suggesting I make his mouth damp before administering medicine.

She takes his temperature with a thermometer that measures from the forehead. It's not extremely accurate, she says, so she takes the temperature on both temples and averages the two numbers. Dave's temp is about 104°F. She suggests we wipe down his body with cool water and apply lotion to make him feel better. The feeling of lotion on damp skin will make his body feel cooler.

"Would you like me to show you how I do it?" she asks.

"Please!" I respond.

Molly is so patient and respectful with Dave. Margaret, Patrick, and I watch her like she's a ballerina performing a solo to a song she's passionate about.

She demonstrates how to roll Dave on his side. While I hold him in position, she cools his back with a washcloth and lotion. We gently roll him back, then she takes each limb and performs the same ritual. He feels cooler already. She is gentle and engaged with each step she takes.

Since Dave has had the catheter, I haven't had much reason to pull down the covers and look at his body. He. Is. So. Skinny. Now that he has purged so much liquid from his cells, his body is gaunt.

Molly loves that we're using the cotton sheet and the gently spinning ceiling fan right over the bed to help keep Dave comfortable. She asks if we have any other questions and whether there's anything else she can do. I can't think of anything. She hugs me, grabs her backpack off the floor, and leaves.

Soon after, Tom arrives at about 10:30 a.m. We all secretly wonder if Dave will pop up the way he did when Patrick and Bobby entered the room. We know it's unlikely since Dave has been on haloperidol and increased fentanyl.

Tom walks into the room and shouts out, "How's my airman doing?" and then takes the pink chair nearest Dave. I hope if Dave is waiting for Tom, he can hear his voice. I offer Tom coffee and banana bread like I have a dozen times when he's come to the house to have coffee with Dave. Tom talks 80 percent of the time, telling stories of how he met Dave, how they went on a boy's bucket-list trip, and about current events. I offer to give him alone time with Dave. He seems to be more comfortable with us in the room. After an hour or so he leaves.

We all secretly wonder if Dave will leave us now.

The rest of the day is essentially uneventful, but busy, nonetheless. Dave receives medicine at 1, 5, 9, and 11 a.m. and

1, 5, 9, and 11 p.m. In between meds, I continue to apply warm and cold compresses to Dave's neck and head. It seems some of the swelling has gone down. His forehead is so smooth, and I wonder where the deep lines that he's had as long as I have known him have gone. *Why is his forehead so smooth?* I wonder over and over, my OCD never letting go. He seems cooler since Molly applied lotion. I repeat the process occasionally, both to comfort Dave and to comfort myself.

Shortly after noon, my friend who's putting together the memorial video sends me the first draft. I dread watching this and go down to the basement so no one will hear me cry. This is the furthest I've been from Dave in weeks. I'm surprisingly unemotional watching the video. It's as if I'm watching someone else's project that needs to be reviewed and critiqued. I have supplied 95 percent of the pictures and instructed which songs should be in the background. My friend, Nora's husband, has done a wonderful job, and he's not surprised when I have a punch list of changes to be made.

I also send him one more picture, instructing him that it must be the last picture of the video. It's a picture of the blue butterfly in the Lucite block that Dave gave me so many years ago. No one at the memorial will understand why this picture appears, but I will. Margaret and Patrick will too. During the many hours we've spent crying, laughing, worrying, and sitting in silence, I have told them the story of the blue butterfly.

When I'm not performing some nursing task, I sit next to Dave and constantly touch him. Stroke him. Whisper to him. Tell him I love him. Tell him he's the best thing that ever happened to me. God, I hope he hears me. I stroke his hair, I stroke his face, still wondering why he no longer has creases in his forehead. I stroke his arms. I stroke his chest. I lay his hand on my leg so I can feel him constantly. I hope he can feel it. *Please know that I am here for you and I will never leave your side.* Occasionally, he twitches, and we never know the cause.

Dave appears to be comfortable for the rest of the day. Molly emptied the urine bag in the morning. The urine continues to drain into the bag, and little by little it's getting darker in color.

After the 9 p.m. meds, Patrick and Margaret leave the bedroom so I can try to sleep for two hours before the 11 p.m. alarm goes off. I turn off the lamps except for the small one by Dave's side of the bed. I listen to how loud his breathing has become. It's really not snoring, but it's comparable to the sound of a snore. I feel strongly that something will happen tonight. Over the last few days, I have often whispered to Dave that I will be okay . . . that I have many people who will take care of me. I don't believe any of this, but I continue to tell him in case that's what is holding him here.

I know this is my husband's body beside me, but it is changing rapidly. The bones in his face have become prominent as the dehydration has caused his face to get thinner. I check below the covers every so often and touch the soft, brown hair on his warm belly. He used to love when I would run my fingers through his belly hair. We've both been curious why the hair on his head turned gray in his thirties but his belly hair is still brown now that he's a seventy-year-old man. His stomach is so sunken in that I can feel his organs.

At 10 p.m. I decide it's not worth going to sleep before his next dose. I'm struggling to keep my eyes open and decide to give him his meds at 10:45. I'm sure fifteen minutes early won't make a difference.

I reluctantly put the earplugs in my ears. I'm afraid with this level of exhaustion I won't hear him if something changes. I doze off shortly after 11.

21

Sunday, October 29

$\mathcal{T}$ he earplugs I've been using are for swimmers, so they completely mold to the inner ear. I abruptly wake up when I hear a change in Dave's breathing. Yanking the earplugs out, I rip out the little baby hairs around my ears that have stuck to them. I look at my watch. It's 12:20 a.m. and I notice a definite change in Dave's breathing. He doesn't have that snore sound anymore. He inhales and takes two short exhales; it sounds more like a frog croaking.

Dave is dying. It hits me square in the face. Dave is dying.

I sob.

Oh Dave! I love you; I love you so much. My Bumpy, I love you so much are some of the words I whisper.

I feel Margaret come in and rub my back. Based on my behavior, she must assume Dave has either passed or is in the process.

The minutes tick by and I can't understand why Dave hasn't stopped breathing.

I desperately want him to stop breathing because it sounds like he's working too hard.

I desperately don't want him to stop breathing because I don't want him to leave me.

Margaret moves to the pink chair when we realize this process may take some time. She asks me if she should call Patrick . . . I tell her no.

I forgo Dave's 1 a.m. meds, assuming his death is imminent. I cry. I caress him. I continue to tell him how much I
love him. By 2:20 a.m. I start to worry that Dave could be in
pain but is unable to show it. I question whether I should give
him his medication, and I remember Molly saying words to the
effect of, "When in doubt . . . do. At the end, no one will question if you gave Dave more morphine because you were afraid
he was in pain." The primary objective is no pain for him . . . a
peaceful death.

I want to do everything right.

Using the dim light of the small lamp on Dave's nightstand,
I administer gentle squirts of the syringe into the sides of his
cheeks so the meds run down his throat or absorb through his
tissue. Only seconds after I do, Dave sounds like he's gagging.

"Margaret! I think he's choking!"

I grab him by his left shoulder and roll his body towards
me. His body is as heavy as a rock. While his head is on its side,
he still seems to be gagging.

I cry out, "Margaret! Oh my God, I've fucked up his death!"

*I am visibly shaken. I don't know what to do. I've done every-
thing right up until now. **Will this be my third mistake?** How could
I have made a mess of things now? I've been so careful. Oh God,
please no!*

Margaret knows I will never forgive myself if this is the
moment that Dave dies. During an extremely long minute,
Dave's gagging stops and his breathing returns to its previous
rhythm.

Inhale. Two croaky exhales.

Inhale. Two croaky exhales.

Minutes feel like hours.

Margaret remains in the pink chair while I am in the position I feel like I have been living in for weeks: immediately to
Dave's right, my left arm wrapped above him so I can stroke
his head, my right hand on his arm or chest. I have positioned

Dave's hand on my leg. I don't know if he can feel this at all, but I still want as many points of contact as I can have without hurting him.

Occasionally I drift to sleep for ten minutes at a time, then open my eyes and see Margaret is doing the same.

Hours pass.

Patrick arrives sometime after the sun comes up. We explain to him what has been occurring since 12:20 a.m. He assumes his position in the pink chair next to his father and takes Dave's hand. He has been holding Dave's hand almost continuously since he arrived nearly a week ago. Margaret moves to the third position, in the dining room chair at Dave's feet.

The three of us . . . never . . . let . . . go.

I message Molly at 7:38 a.m. and ask her what time she starts work. I explain to her how Dave's breathing changed during the night. She says she will be here within the hour.

Sadie is at the foot of the bed near me when Molly arrives at 8:18 a.m. The door to the room is closer to my side of the bed, so Molly walks past the foot of the bed around to Dave's side, just as she did yesterday. Again she talks to Dave as if he is awake. She addresses the rest of us softly and with calmness, yet energy pours off her. Her presence alone is able to relieve some of the quiet tension that has been building in the room.

There is one soul in the room that is not comforted when Molly lays hands on Dave. It is Sadie. When Molly leans in to touch Dave, Sadie turns her head to her and growls. Sadie has done so well for weeks with all the coming and going of people. This is the first time we've heard her growl since all this started. Her eyes are big, her head is low, her ears even lower.

Molly talks quietly to Sadie and extends her hand gently. Sadie growls again, not in an aggressive manner but in a way that tells us she knows something is wrong. Sadie knows Dave is leaving us. Molly, who is a dog person, says to her,

"That's okay Sadie, we don't have to be friends today." As I calm Sadie, she turns her head away from Molly and gently rests it on the bed.

Molly tells us Dave's breathing is normal for the stage he is at; it is part of the dying process. Dave is not suffering. He is not gasping for air. His body does not need the amount of air it once did, much like the way he reduced his food and water intake. She tells me there may come a time when as much as a minute or a minute and a half could pass between breaths.

"Is this the death rattle I've heard so much about?" I ask her.

She says it is, but because we've been giving Dave medication to minimize mucus, it will not sound so rattly.

I tell her how I thought I'd killed Dave by choking him with the medication last night. How ironic, the thought of accidentally killing a hospice patient. Molly demonstrates how Dave might be able to tolerate receiving meds more easily. She offers to do anything before she leaves, and I ask her to swab Dave's mouth. She does it so much better than me; I'm afraid of hurting him.

I want to do everything right.

Molly leaves at 9 a.m. and tells me to go outside and take ten deep breaths. I just smile at her. I have no intention of going outside.

At 9:14 a.m. I receive her text: "Ten breaths outside . . . maybe five if ten feels like too much."

We have a door in our bedroom that leads to our back porch. We've been keeping it open during the day because the days have been beautiful with low humidity and it's the only way any of us see the sunshine. I go to the back porch, still in eyesight of Dave, and take some deep breaths.

At 11:45 a.m. I send a text to Bobby: "Will you stop by for a prayer? I believe Dave will be leaving us today." He replies that he will arrive about 1:30 p.m.

As the hours continue, I look at my watch and announce when it has been six hours . . . eight hours . . . ten hours . . . that Dave has been breathing this horrible froggy-sounding breath.

When Bobby arrives, it's been thirteen hours since Dave's breathing changed. Not many words are said. We pray and Bobby leaves.

I have barely moved a muscle since the middle of the night, only to grab Dave's medicine, visit the bathroom, and take the quick breaths outside that Molly suggested. Patrick and Margaret remain in their seats, the pink chair and the dining chair, respectively. Margaret retrieves cool washcloths for me when I need them so I don't have to leave the bed. More than once, the temperature of Dave's body has cycled between burning up and cooling down.

I have rearranged Dave's arm on my leg, his hand cupping my foot, trying to find the most natural position for his arm to rest. When I'm on the bed, I'm touching him . . . stroking him . . . whispering to him. I was never this physically affectionate during most of the years of our marriage, but for the last week, I've been absolutely magnetized to him. I can't stop touching him.

I don't understand how Dave's heart is so strong. How could his body go through such turmoil and his heart be this strong?

The hours continue.

It's unspoken, but no one wants to leave the room. We all want to be there for Dave's final breath.

I continue with all the nursing tasks—meds, washcloths, lotion. I lovingly continue all the wifely tasks—hugging, crying, touching, and telling my Bumpy how much I love him.

At 3:38 p.m., Margaret leaves the room, for what I don't know.

The exhale that Dave makes sounds dreadful, then there is a long pause. Patrick and I hold our breath . . . Dave sucks in air . . . Patrick and I breathe quickly, glancing at each other. We feel like we dodged a bullet.

Dave takes a couple more breaths and the same thing happens again. Froggy exhale . . . silence for at least thirty seconds . . . Patrick and I hold our breath . . . I'm sure this is it . . . my heart beats faster . . . Patrick and I glance at each other . . . I'm terrified . . . this can't really be happening now . . . three years we've been on the cancer train . . .

Dave sucks in air . . . Patrick and I breathe.

I can't imagine how much longer this can go on. It's now been fifteen and a half hours since this shift in breathing started.

Dave takes a couple more breaths . . .

The froggy double exhale comes out . . .

Waiting . . . waiting . . . waiting . . . waiting . . . waiting . . .
. . . nothing.

Dave takes his last breath at 3:41 p.m.

Dave has died.

I wrap my arms around his head and cry hard. I call out his name. "Bumpy . . . Bumpy . . . I love you Bumpy . . . I'm going to miss you so much . . . I love you so much!" The world feels over. Like someone doused out the sun forever.

Margaret rushes back in. I am wrapped around Dave, no longer afraid of crushing his frail body. Patrick is in the pink chair and holding Dave's hand; he is crying. Margaret is in the chair at the end of the bed, holding Dave's cold feet with her head bowed down. The three of us grieve in our designated positions.

We continue to grieve over Dave's body when my phone rings exactly eleven minutes after Dave died. *Who could be calling me? Who could have such bad timing?* I look at the number. I think it might be hospice. It's Shirelle, the nurse navigator who reminds me of Mary Poppins. As soon as she says hello, I recognize her soothing accent. She is calling to see how things are going with hospice and asks if we are getting everything we need.

I tell her Dave just died moments ago. She's aghast at her bad timing, but the way she says, "Oh, dear, dear, I am so sorry," reminds me of the day I fell into her arms as she comforted me at the bottom of the front stairs. I tell her I haven't called anyone yet, that it *just* happened. She tells me not to worry about making phone calls; she will take care of it.

Margaret and Patrick leave the room to give me time alone with Dave's body. I continue to cry. I beg to Dave, "Please give me a sign you are okay . . . please give me a sign . . . send me blue butterflies . . . please let me know you are okay."

I run my hands over his whole body. I look at his face. The tumor that has been bright red and growing profusely since July has drained of blood and is now the color of his skin. It's a visual that suggests he's not hurting anymore. No more tumor. No more cancer. No more pain.

Staring at him, I take in how much his face has changed in the last twenty-four hours. The rosy color is gone, replaced by a yellow tinge. The swelling from his face is gone, and I realize just how thin his face has become; his cheekbones are pronounced. His eyes are half closed, so I gently use my fingers to lower his lids all the way. His mouth remains half open as it has been for the last several days. I notice the inside of his mouth appears to have darkened.

We noticed yesterday that Dave's hands and feet were the first to show a temperature change as his circulation slowed. But now, as I slip my hands under the bright-blue sheet, his arms and legs are cold. I run my hands over his chest and protruding ribs, which I've been so afraid of hurting for so many months. My hands, still under the sheet, run up his leg. His thighs are still warm. My hands stop at the diaper. I hope he never knew he was wearing one. I pray if he did, he knew not to feel embarrassed.

My hands push the white undershirt up to just where his ribs start. His belly is so warm, so warm I can't leave it. I know soon his whole body will be cold. I look at his arms lying at his sides and remember how much he liked to lie with both arms propped behind his head. Margaret and Patrick said Dave's dad liked to lie the same way. I consider moving his arms and worry about how soon it will be before his body becomes stiff. I think back to my police academy crime scene class over thirty-five years ago and remember something about rigor mortis setting in and then the body softening again, but I don't remember how long that process takes. I decide to take the chance.

I gently take his left arm. It's no heavier than it was before; he had absolutely no control of his arms when I was cooling them with a washcloth only earlier today. I slowly lift it and bring his fingers just to the edge of his ear. I don't want to force his arm, so I prop a pillow under his elbow to hold it in place. I do the same with his right arm. Now that Dave looks comfortable and his belly is still warm, I take my place. I lie perpendicular to his body, no longer afraid of breaking his bones, and lay my head directly on his bare, warm belly, still being careful to have the sheet just high enough to give him the dignity he deserves.

I grab my phone to scroll through my music, looking for one song, the one we spoke of long ago.

Dave and I speak rather abstractly about music prefer-ences at a funeral. He mentions a song.

"Yes, I love that song . . . the version from Meet Joe Black, *right?" I ask.*

Of course that's the best version, we agree.

Eventually, Dave selects for me all the music to be played at his funeral. He sits at the dining room table with headphones on so I don't have to live through hours of hearing him select songs. On the writing tablet next to the computer, he makes a list of the songs he has chosen. I occasionally peek at the list, asking him one day if he wants all of the music on that list played. I think it some-what ironic since, generally, he doesn't enjoy music the way I do.

He says, "Nah, you don't have to play it all. But this will give you a selection to work with."

But I know there is one song that will definitely be played.

I scroll down the list on my phone. There it is. I close my eyes, my head still on Dave's warm belly as "Somewhere Over the Rainbow" by Israel Kamakawiwo'ole plays. I half sing, half hum, so relieved he is no longer in pain . . . so devastated he is no longer here with me. The song finishes and the next starts.

Go back. Repeat. Play it again. After the second play-through, I stop the music.

I still want to do everything right.

At 4:44 p.m., I message Bobby: "Dave has passed."

At 4:49 p.m., Bobby walks into the room. For me, Bobby is the perfect pastor. He doesn't try to convince me he under-stands why awful things happen to good people. He doesn't say that Dave is in a better place. He doesn't say this is all for the better.

Bobby tells me he loves me; God loves me; God loves Dave. I ask him to promise me Dave is okay. He can't make any prom-ises but tries to give me as much proof as he can by sharing scripture and telling me that Dave is okay now . . . that Dave is better than okay.

Ten minutes later, Molly walks into the room. She exchanges hellos with Bobby before he hugs me and leaves. I can't be more relieved to see that it's Molly and not another nurse. When she hugs me, she holds me with her hand against the back of my head like she did before. Her hugs are so genuine.

She tells me she knows it's silly, but she has to confirm Dave has passed. I understand. I resume my position in the bed next to Dave while Molly pulls out her stethoscope and looks at her wristwatch. She wears a wristwatch and not a fitness watch. I'm almost surprised, but I suppose she likes the second hand.

Time is moving by, but it feels like this is not real. I am here, but not here. This is what the last six weeks have been leading up to. Now it's over. It's like when I was younger and would make big plans for New Year's Eve. I'd buy a new outfit, choose a special guy and a special place, and wear more makeup than usual. I'd make big plans and wait all night for the ten-second countdown. Then, in the blink of an eye, New Year's Eve was over and the New Year was here.

I can see just a sliver of Dave's eyes again. Molly sees me try to lower his lids and explains that his lower lids are pulling away, which is why the top lid is no longer able to cover his eye completely. Dave's mouth remains partially open; it appears the inside of his mouth is now turning black.

Molly offers to wash Dave's body. Although I find it relaxing to watch how tender she is when handling Dave, he is not very dirty or sweaty. She offers to remove the catheter. "Yes! Please do that," I say. "And let's put regular underwear on him." She is more than pleased to help. After Molly removes the catheter, she glides between the bedroom and the bathroom, disposing of the catheter and urine. I notice that his urine has indeed become the color of steeped tea.

At 5:20 p.m. I feel a text come through. I glance at my watch. It's from Tracey. It says only, "Love you," but it comes with the emoji of the smiley face blowing a kiss. She must have heard about Dave's passing from Bobby. She and Jeremy are close friends with Bobby also.

Meanwhile, I open Dave's underwear drawer and look at the old underwear and the new, better-fitting ones I just bought him a couple of weeks ago. I decide on the new ones—the first of many decisions I will make alone. I try to choose between the navy, the red, or the striped ones. The decision seems so important. My OCD kicks in. *Dave, how will I make these little decisions, the ones I obsess over, without you here?* I decide on the blue underwear, assuming I will use the striped ones for his final outfit.

I wiggle them up his legs. Molly and I each take a leg and lift Dave's hips as we pull the underwear up. It's bunched in the back. She knows it needs to be fixed. I love the fact that it's important to her that we fix the bunched-up underwear. If he were alive, it would be uncomfortable.

She asks if I want to change his undershirt. No, I just changed it this morning. Jessica showed me how to take a shirt and cut it up the back, stopping just an inch or two below the neckline so the shirt can be pulled over the head and slipped over the arms, fitting much like a hospital gown would.

Molly pulls the bright-blue sheet up to Dave's waist. His arms are still propped up, and his hands are as close to behind his head as possible. He looks like he's sleeping. Molly asks if there is anything else she can do for me. I tell her no. The funeral home will take about forty-five minutes before they arrive. She won't call them until I want her to. I tell her she can call them now.

As I wait on the bed for the funeral director to arrive, I call Sadie to the room. She jumps onto the bed. It's so odd she is willing, considering she has never cared much for coming onto the bed when Dave and I are both in it. Instead of her usual circling and then lying at the foot, she takes one step closer to

Dave's body. She extends her neck, reaching to sniff his hand. She recoils, turns, and jumps off the bed. She knows. She knows something is different. There is no doubt in my mind a dog knows the difference between dead and alive.

Five minutes after Molly leaves, at 5:43 p.m., I hear another voice in the living room. I peek my head out and see Tracey holding a container of something. I go out to greet her. She stumbles through her words and her eyes are red. She tells me she was making stew when she heard the news, so she threw some in a container and rushed it over for us. She hands me the container; it's still warm. We embrace and cry. I wonder if every time I see someone for the first time after Dave's death I will cry when I hug them. I'm fairly certain the answer is yes. Tracey leaves after the embrace, wiping her eyes as she runs down the stairs.

Margaret and Patrick return to the bedroom with me. At 6:13 p.m. I hear someone on the front porch. It's the funeral director and his assistant. Dave doesn't need me by his side anymore, and it is my responsibility to greet them. I introduce myself as Dave's wife and tell them to follow me. I wonder how these two gentlemen, certainly both near or over the age of seventy, will be able to carry my husband down the stairs. They follow me to the bedroom, and I slide across the bed to the position I have maintained for eight days.

The thinner man does almost all the talking. I look at how well-dressed he is and wonder what he was doing before he got the phone call. Was he watching football on TV and then the phone rang with the voice on the other end telling him to pick up a body? Did he then go into his bedroom to put on his suit, and was it all pressed and ready to jump into? I notice his nametag. His last name is Smith. Right . . . I remember he introduced himself as Bart Smith moments ago, but I didn't make the connection. Now I see why his suit, shirt, and tie are so well-coordinated. The name of the funeral home is Smith.

He is one of the owners. I don't think he says anything of consequence, but I acknowledge him as he speaks.

I quickly glance at the quiet one. He's much heavier. He's going to struggle on those stairs. He's wearing a simple, clean suit, but it's obvious he's the assistant. They both momentarily leave the house to bring in a gurney. Then they realize they won't be able to negotiate the turns of the doorway into the bedroom. The heavier man goes back to the car to bring in a board with straps so they can slide Dave onto it and carry him to the gurney they left in the hallway—the hallway where I flung the jar of ointment. I maintain my position on the bed, telling Bart I am not leaving the room, or the bed for that matter. I am not asking a question; I am making a statement.

I share with him my concerns about Dave's arms. Bart must be looking at Dave's arms over his head and wondering why he's propped up like he's watching a ball game. I tell him that's how Dave likes to sleep.

I reach for Dave's right arm and gasp when I realize it has stiffened. *Oh God, did I screw up?* Bart says not to worry. He starts manipulating Dave's left arm. The entire time he does, I am petrified I might hear Dave's bone or joint snap. I would be truly horrified! I know this is only Dave's body and Dave is no longer inside, but it would be my fault if his bone were to break. Thankfully, it does not.

Both arms are lowered to Dave's sides. I can see his hands are completely devoid of color. They look like a bad wax museum mannequin. I can't take my eyes off his hands. I pick one up and look at his nail beds and cuticles. They aren't pink anymore and they resemble a plastic doll. I am transfixed by the changes in Dave's body over the last hour.

When the heavier man brings the board to the bed, he slides it under Dave. I follow Bart's lead, securing Dave's arms. They keep flopping, so I hold his right one in place until it can be secured with a buckle.

"I want the blue sheet back," I tell them.

They cover Dave's body with a white sheet and pull my bright-blue one out from below, so Dave's body is never without a cover. They pull the board off the bed and carry Dave to the gurney waiting in the hallway. The gurney is wheeled to the front door, where they stop in case I want to say goodbye.

They don't know me. They don't know that I have control issues and that I will not relinquish control until Dave is secured in the car. I imagine most wives don't get this involved in stabilizing and securing the body of their late husband, but I am different. *I am Dave's number-one advocate . . . his number-one fan . . . his person . . . his Snookums.*

A green blanket embroidered with the name SMITH covers Dave up to his chin. I cradle Dave's face and tell my Bumpy how much I love him and will miss him.

The men pull the blanket over Dave's face and secure it. Margaret holds the door open while they roll the gurney out to the porch. They have sixteen stairs before they get to the ground. Bart takes the bottom. When they realize how difficult this will be, Margaret shimmies past them to get behind Bart and guide his steps. She places both of her hands on his back to secure him. I assume the position to the right side of Dave . . . the same position I have been in nearly constantly, not only for the last eight days but for essentially the last twenty-one years.

I am shocked at the weight of everything and so afraid the heavy man will not be able to support his end. He lifts his end and sets the casters on each step, one step at a time. We make it to the landing. I know he can't wait to get to flat ground. My mind imagines the gurney falling through the air. That cannot happen.

I need to do everything right.

We finally get to the bottom of the stairs, and they slide the gurney into the car. I'm surprised the car resembles an

SUV more than it does a hearse. I wonder if my neighbors are watching. I wonder if they realize Dave has died.

The heavy man starts the car as Bart comes over to talk to me. I have no idea what he says. When Bart gets in the car, Margaret comes over to hold me.

Letting the tears flow, I keep repeating, "It's never going to get better . . . it's never going to get better."

It's 6:35 p.m. when they pull out of the driveway. I break away from Margaret so I can walk to the edge of the street to watch the car pull away. I can't believe Dave is gone. I watch them drive down the street . . . stop at the intersection . . . make a left turn to return to the funeral home. I remain in place, still knowing I can catch a glimpse of the car as it passes between the first and second house from the corner.

It's over.

The last three years . . . the doctors, the research, the shakes, the bucket-list trips, the hyperbaric oxygen therapy, the massages, the immunotherapy, the chemotherapy, the radiation, the three-hour drives to the doctor, the scans, the worry, the stress, the rollercoaster, the cancer train . . .

It's over.

More importantly, the last twenty-two years of conversation, the hugs, the companionship, the love, the support, my husband . . . my buddy . . . my partner . . . my friend . . . my person . . . my teammate on a two-person team . . . is no longer here. I just can't believe it. In the last two weeks, I've been so focused on Dave having the quiet, pain-free death he wanted that I've never really thought about what happens when he's gone.

I walk inside with Margaret and Patrick and head straight to the bedroom. The bed has only a fitted sheet and some pillows on it. The bright-blue sheet was tossed to the side. That sheet is the last thing that touched Dave's body. I wrap it around mine and curl up on the bed. The void is massive. He's no longer here for me to take care of. He's no longer here to take care of me. I feel so empty.

The rest of the night passes in a fog. I walk around, probably resembling a zombie more than a woman. I don't remember whether I've eaten. I was about to call Megan when I found out Patrick had already called her. Ultimately, she calls me and we cry together.

Weeks ago, Dave and I made a list off his phone of people he wanted notified of his passing. Margaret, Patrick, and I break up the list and go to our respective corners of the house to make phone calls.

When all is done, I go into our bedroom. There are a dozen pillows around the room and on the bed we were using for Dave's comfort, all the medical supplies we used are lying around, and the pink chair and the dining chair are still in place. I pull most of the pillows off the bed, making sure to leave the one Dave's head was last on. I float the bright-blue sheet onto the bed. It's a queen-size sheet on a king-size bed, but that's insignificant. I fluff the comforter and place it atop the sheet. I put Sloth on Dave's side, where Sloth lives. "My spirit animal," Dave would say.

I announce I'm going to bed. I toss a sleeping pill into my mouth and position myself diagonally, my feet on my side of the bed and my head on Dave's. This is exactly how I used to sleep before I married Dave—on a diagonal, usually with a dog at the foot of the bed. This is how I will sleep again—with my head on Dave's side of the bed . . . Sloth tucked into my chest.

Surprisingly, I fall asleep easier than expected. I wake only once during the night. Quickly remembering the circumstances of my life, I beg for my brain to shut off. I fall back to sleep quickly.

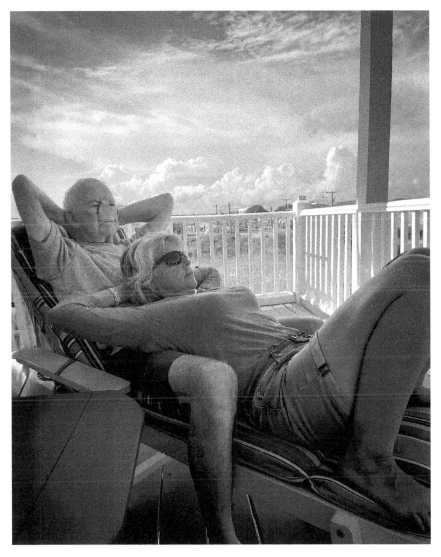

September 10, 2023: A contemplative moment

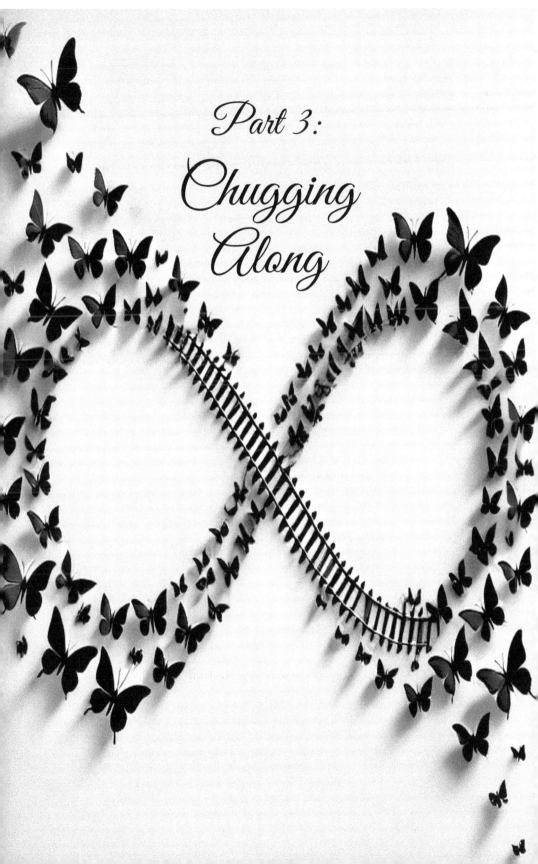

Part 3:

Chugging Along

Monday, October 30

$\mathcal{U}$pon waking, the first thing I do is cry. I knew mornings would be hardest for me. It's that moment when you wake from sleep, just before you realize where you are in your life, and then it all floods in. That's the moment the tears start.

I brush my teeth, walk to the kitchen, make coffee, sit on the couch . . . and cry again. Margaret is staying at the house through the funeral and the memorial service. Claire will join us in a couple of days. There is no one in the world, other than Dave, I want near me right now more than Margaret and Claire. They both have healing spirits and are incredibly wise, and they know how to float through the house to offer companionship when needed and become invisible when necessary.

The first order of business is to get my little Sadie out for a walk. It's now been weeks since Joan has been walking Sadie. She needs some normalcy, and I should probably get some fresh air. My normal life consists of lots of outdoor activity, and I haven't left the house for eight days.

As I walk Sadie on the beach, I look at the beautiful ocean with the sun glimmering off the waves. I think back to the walk Dave and I took on this beach nine years ago when we first found this island. We had no idea what was in store for us. I feel the pain of losing him well up inside me. It's been less than twenty-four hours since he died. This time yesterday, he was breathing, making that awful sound, and I was lying beside him waiting for him to take his last breath. I look at my watch and see it's 11:15 a.m. I think to myself, *Just try to make it till noon. When the days are too overwhelming, break them down into hours and minutes.*

When I return from the walk, I focus on tasks. The first is to get my bedroom in order. I pull all the pillowcases off a dozen pillows lying around the room. Of course, the yellow pillow that was under Dave and the bright-blue sheet will remain untouched. The pink chair goes back to its place in the living room, the dining chair goes back to its corner in my bedroom, and the mountain of used tissues that dried my tears go in the garbage.

I walk to the bathroom and burst into tears. In my mind's eye, I suddenly see Dave lying on the bathroom floor, toilet seat in the air and him curled up. I look around the room and see all his belongings on the vanity. Dave liked to keep his daily toiletries out where he could see them. I was forever tossing them in the drawer. It was an ongoing battle . . . one I know I will miss. Now I don't want to move anything of his. I knew this would happen, which is why I happily organized all his stuff when he was still alive. I knew I wouldn't want to disturb anything after he was gone. I see his new electric toothbrush, used only twice, next to all his manhole covers and nose-care toiletries. I cry some more.

The one thing I want to get rid of is everything related to cancer. I pour the liquid opioids down the drain and toss all the pills and patches into a baggie for disposal at the local police department. I hate cancer. I just fucking hate it. The medical supply company calls and says they will come get the oxygen today. I'm anxious to get it out of the house.

Next task is to select Dave's final outfit. I pull out the blue shirt I bought him for his brother and sister-in-law's fiftieth wedding anniversary. He loved that shirt! It's a simple button-down in comfortable fabric that has blue sharks on it. It looked great on him! That was the only thing Dave and I discussed about his final outfit. We didn't really discuss it at all, but I asked him if he thought the shirt would be a good idea. He wasn't interested in picking out the clothes himself. He either trusted his wife would make the right choice or didn't really care.

I pull out seven pairs of shorts and lay them next to the shirt. This pair is too matchy-matchy . . . he didn't really like this pair . . . that one's too casual . . . this one's too black. I settle on a pair of tan, dressy shorts.

It's an easy decision for the footwear. Dave raved about the sandals I bought him this summer and said they were the best sandals he ever had.

I pull out his whitest undershirt and head for the underwear drawer. I recall that yesterday I saved the striped ones for today. No, they're not right. I think back to when I joked with Dave about how sexy he would look in the striped underwear, but I know he was more of a solids kind of guy. I grab the brick-red underwear that's more his speed. *I have his shirt, shorts, tee, underwear . . . I need a belt!* I grab his casual belt, the one without the holes. It's the only one he wore since he could adjust it to any size.

Then I see his watch on the dresser. It's just a simple Timex, but he thought it ran great. He used to have a leather strap, but when he was losing weight he was having difficulty making it comfortable; it kept spinning around his wrist. I took the watch to the watch store and bought him a black band that has an adjustable Velcro strap. He thought it was the best thing ever!

Next, I write instructions to the person who will be dressing my husband for the last time:

- Top two buttons of shirt left unbuttoned
- Undershirt tucked into underwear
- Watch on left wrist
- Shirt untucked

My OCD is still at play. I need to do everything right.

I will be the only person who sees Dave "in the box," as I've been calling it. We discussed this back when we planned his funeral. Dave didn't want people gawking at him. I didn't think anyone would gawk. The funny thing is, no one ever described Dave as "the guy without a nose." Hardly anyone in the world knows someone who doesn't have a nose, but people looked at Dave with his beige manhole cover we designed years ago and just didn't notice. He was never defined by having cancer or not having a nose. I don't know of anyone else who could pull that off.

When we planned the funeral, Dave and I decided it would be only family and close friends at the funeral and cemetery. The rest of the world could join us at the memorial service the next day. I also told Dave I needed to see him in the box. Maybe it was because my father died when I was ten years old and I didn't get to see him because he had a closed casket. Maybe it was because I really needed to see this through. Number-one advocate . . . number-one caregiver . . . I need to make sure my person is put to rest just the way we wanted. I need to make sure everything is done right.

And maybe I knew I would need to see him to believe he is actually gone.

I also needed to put Buddy Bear in the casket. Buddy Bear is a stuffed bear that was given to Dave by his uncle Buddy when Dave was a baby. The bear had been mended by his mother, with particular attention given to the nose . . . rather ironic actually. Margaret tells me their brother Tom used to poke the bear's nose to torment little brother Dave. Flo, Dave's mother, tied a Christmas ribbon around the bear's neck after she mended him. Buddy Bear has sat in a position of prominence in our bedroom for as long as I have known Dave, who made it clear that he wants Buddy Bear in the box.

I also want to put one of Dave's hats in the box. It's the gray, floppy hat with the logo of our favorite coffee shop. I swear Dave was a walking billboard for Jeremy and Tracey's shop over the years because he wore their hats, T-shirts, and sweatshirts all around the country on our bucket-list trips.

For months, in the back of my head, I've been thinking about putting in the "three-carrot" ring Dave gave me. Being the prankster he is, one year, back in the early days before we were even married, he said he'd bought me a three-carat ring. *What?!* It turned out the ring was plastic and had three plastic two-inch carrots sticking out of it. I thought for sure I had it in my keep-it box. A couple of weeks ago, Dave and I looked through the box, much the way we did his, and I was quite disturbed to not be able to find the ring. I can't imagine where it is, as that would be the only place I would have put it. I don't even know where to start looking. I guess I'll just place Buddy Bear and the hat in the box.

Dave's wedding band remains on a chain around my neck . . . I still need to get a stronger chain as Dave suggested.

I gather the clothes and instructions for the funeral home. I also need to go there to sign the death certificate and confirm it has the correct information. I ask Margaret and Patrick to go with me. It would be way too easy to make a mistake now. I'm trying to focus on tasks, but I still feel like I'm in a movie. This just can't be my life . . . without Dave.

Just getting behind the wheel feels strange. I haven't driven in weeks, but the first stop is to the coffee shop so I can get my usual drink. I'm likely to see some of our favorite people there, including the girls who loved Dave and came to visit him when he couldn't get out of the house. On the way, I see an object in the road in the distance. As I near it, I realize it's a turtle. Being an avid animal lover, I swerve to the side of the road, put the car in park, turn on the flashers, and run down the middle of the road so cars realize there's something to watch out for. I notice the turtle's direction of travel, scoop him up, and escort him about twenty feet off the road in the direction he was traveling. I comment to my passengers, Margaret and Patrick, that this is only the second turtle I've seen in the last eight years since Dave and I moved here. Margaret, who's a huge believer in signs from the universe, mentions that a turtle is very "sloth-like." I chuckle. I would love to believe Dave is sending signs, but I don't think a turtle in the road is a sign.

We arrive at the coffee shop and my companions wait in the car. I step out of the car, shut the door, and hear music playing on the speaker outside the building. It's "Somewhere Over the Rainbow." It's not my favorite version, but it's *the* song. I open the back door where Patrick is sitting and tell him and Margaret to listen to the song as I stand there crying. I stand at the car long enough to collect myself before going into the building to get my coffee and share some more tears with Ashley.

When I return to the car, Margaret starts talking about signs. She wonders whether the sloth-like turtle had crossed our path to slow us down just enough so that when I got out of the car, I heard *the* song. "Margaret," I say, "there's a thing in the law they call 'clear and convincing evidence.' That's not clear and convincing." She's baffled that I'm such a nonbeliever and jokes that her poor brother is up there sending down signs. It's only his first day on the job, but I'm still skeptical.

We continue on our drive to the funeral home and see some cars stopped in the road ahead of us. A small dog is running around the street. Being used to jumping out of the car to rescue loose dogs, I have a dog leash within an arm's distance. I again swerve to the side of the road, park the car, and put the flashers on, this time grabbing the leash. I run across the road and spend several minutes with others trying to get this little five-pound scrappy dog to safety. I'm satisfied when he runs away from the direction of the road towards some secluded houses where he might live, but if not, at least he won't get hit by a car. I walk back to the car and get in. Before Margaret has a chance to say anything, I say, "Shut up Margaret." We all laugh. I tell her I want blue butterflies. She tells me it's only his first day and to cut him some slack.

Dave, are you really okay? I would do anything to know you are, but I don't want to believe just for the sake of believing. I don't want to believe just to make myself feel better. I won't feel better unless you're okay.

The funeral home confirms the time of the cemetery ceremony. Dave will be buried in a veteran's cemetery, and they only do burials at 10 a.m., noon, and 2 p.m., so all planning is based on this time confirmation.

Now that the time is set in stone, an onslaught of work ensues. Thank God I have Margaret and Tracey. Between the three of us, we iron out details.

The number of people traveling for this funeral would be staggering to Dave. I used to tell him there would be "standing room only," but he insisted that people have jobs, kids, and responsibilities and that not everyone who wanted to come would be able to. I asked him, "Would you go to [so-and-so's] funeral?" He replied, "Yes, I would, but that's different." Dave is unaware of the lasting impact he has made on so many lives. He is . . . was . . . a humble man.

When it's dinner time, Ashley asks if she can stop by with soup. The outside temperature has dropped several degrees. Magically, she appears with warm chicken noodle soup, the ultimate comfort food. I pour us three bowls, then Margaret, Patrick, and I sit at the dining table to eat.

I have survived my first day without Dave.

At night, I sit and work on my journal for hours. I've been stressed all day, and my OCD brain is fixated on the fact that I have not written anything down for days. As much as I thought I wouldn't . . . couldn't . . . forget anything, as much as I thought every minute was burned into my brain, the whole experience is now running together. I start piecing events together with texts and my security cameras.

I turn off the light just before 2 a.m. My brain never stops working.

23

Tuesday, October 31

I tossed, turned, and slept horribly last night and was exhausted when I got up for the day. I'm still sleeping diagonally and with the bright-blue sheet and the yellow pillow. It gives me the tiniest bit of comfort to know these fabrics were the last to touch Dave's body. I just wish we'd picked a more comfortable pillow for him! I hate this pillow. I like soft, squishy pillows. We used this one for Dave because it was firm and he looked more comfortable on it when he was lying in the same position for many hours at a time. For now, it's my preferred pillow, because it was his.

The cleaning people are coming today, so I rise and shower. My first errand is to run by the coffee shop to drop off a house key for Tracey. She's handling the refreshments after the funeral and the memorial and will have everything set up at the house when the family returns. I doubt she realizes what a huge relief she's providing me by handling this.

The girls in the coffee shop have been writing messages on Dave's and my cups for weeks now. They went over the top with adorableness when they wrote messages on Dave's cup. But they often put a sweet one on mine too. Today, one of our favorite baristas writes, "We love you."

Tracey is not at the shop, but Jeremy is in his office. It's the first time I've seen him since Dave's death. The last time I saw Jeremy, Dave was trying to assuage Jeremy's tears by playfully suggesting a BJ. We hug for a long time and share some tears. Our conversation is fairly brief. Jeremy is one of two friends who will be speaking at Dave's memorial. The other is Colonel Tom.

I leave the shop to continue with my errands. Next stop is the food pantry. I have about eight-and-a-half-dozen nutrition shakes I will no longer need. Maybe someone else can benefit from them. I give them the shakes, cans of organic coconut milk, bottles of Norwegian cod liver oil, and bags of fresh beets, all ingredients from Dave's magical shakes. The volunteer at the food pantry is grateful for my donation.

Third stop is the funeral parlor to fax the documents for Dave's headstone. The headstone is fairly conventional, as Dave is being buried at a VA cemetery. It will have his name, date of birth, rank, and branch of service as well as the conflict Dave served in. I can personalize the stone with twenty-five characters. Had I known this, I would have obsessed over what to write for months. But I had about twenty-four hours to come up with something. It actually took less than ten minutes.

FLY HIGH BUMPY

Perfect.

I fax the paperwork from the funeral home to the VA and continue on to repairing a necklace. There's no urgency to repair the chain, but I just had it repaired a month ago and when I picked it up, it broke again. More importantly, this is one of Dave's gifts to me from one of our trips.

We're in Hendersonville, North Carolina. The idea of spending the month of August in the mountains instead of at our hot, crowded beach is very appealing. This is the first year we decide to leave the beach in the summer months, and it's only for two weeks. Just like usual, mid-week, Dave goes off one day and buys me a present. It's an

antique-looking necklace we'd seen in a store window, a
chain with a dragonfly pendant.

Staying focused on tasks, I head to get my allergy shot. When I walk in, I give my name to the person behind the desk, and as usual she asks for my birthdate. Though I've been reciting my birthdate to her once a week for months, I stutter and start to give Dave's birthdate out of habit. We've visited so many doctors over the last few years, and with my brain being in such a fog now, it actually takes me a second to recite my own.

My last errand is a manicure. Nancy, my manicurist, knows Dave has been sick. She hugs me the minute I walk into the shop. While she does my nails, I look around at the happy ladies getting manicures and pedicures and think, *You never know what's going on in someone's life . . . I'm sure no one would look at me and think, "That lady looks like she just lost her husband."*

Finally, I head in the direction of home. Moments before I turn onto my dead-end street, my phone rings. The caller ID shows it's Dr. Thorn. Under normal circumstances, before Dave's death, I would know the caller was actually someone from Dr. Thorn's office calling to change an appointment or confirm something. After all, top-notch surgeons don't make patient phone calls. Today, I know differently. Via the patient portal, I'd sent the obituary that Dave and I wrote to Dr. Thorn, Dr. Shilo, and Mario. I have no doubt who is on the other end of that phone.

"Brent," I answer. I suppose I caught him off guard. He stammers a bit with condolences.

This is not the first personal tragedy I've shared with Dr. Thorn. During the three years he was our surgeon, his wife, also a medical professional, lost a baby at full term. I wrote a letter of sympathy to him, and he responded by saying he was able to use the grace and strength he saw in Dave and me to help him and his wife get through their tragedy. His reply affected me deeply. I didn't even realize Dave and I exhibited grace and strength. I was just trying to put one foot in front of the other and make my husband healthy.

Ultimately, they had another pregnancy and gave birth to a boy earlier this year. We bought some adorable baby bibs and brought them with us to one of our appointments this past spring.

Two and a half weeks before Dave's death, I sent a letter to our doctors. I knew after Dave died, I wouldn't feel like writing it. This is an excerpt that addressed Dr. Thorn, who was never pretentious and always identified himself by his first name:

> You remember our first visit, I was a bit surprised that we weren't seeing Dr. Z? And then you called us on a Tuesday night to give us the results of some tests. I was a bit perturbed that we were shifting gears . . . getting a new doctor when it wasn't my choice. Our conversation was a bit testy, on my end, but we made the "Jersey connection" and you told me we needed to put Dr. Z in the past . . . move forward . . . you would do the best you possibly could to take care of my husband.
>
> Your take-charge, yet not condescending attitude resonated with me. I liked you from that moment on. I am so thankful you became our doctor! I would travel far and wide for your opinion. It's rare that a surgeon has a bedside manner like yours. I think you're brilliant, sensitive, and caring. I will always be thankful we crossed paths with you on this awful cancer journey.

As I speak with Dr. Thorn, I describe how awful the last eight days of Dave's life were. I go into detail, figuring as a surgeon he must know what happens when someone is close to death. But maybe he doesn't. If someone dies on the operating table, it's a sudden death. If someone dies in hospice care, he never hears about it. So maybe someone who deals with life and death day in and day out doesn't actually know what happens in those last eight days.

For that matter, maybe most doctors don't know. And maybe most nurses don't know—hospice nurses excluded, of course. So maybe, just maybe, nearly the entire world—thanatologists excluded—doesn't know what happens when a person is nearing a "natural" death from the perspective of a caregiver.

As I describe how awful the last eight days were, I cry profusely. Dr. Thorn patiently listens until I'm done. He tells me that Dave was a one-in-a-million guy and that meeting him changed him both as a person and as a surgeon. He says that meeting me has set the bar for what a supportive wife and advocate can be and that knowing us as a couple has changed his life forever. He is very clear that if he can ever, ever do anything for me, to call his office. Knowing this young, brilliant surgeon the way I do, I know he means it.

When I return home, Nora's husband sends me the next version of Dave's memorial video. It's getting better but I want more edits. I'm sorry. I know I'm being demanding with my friend's generosity. But he knows me well enough to know that my expectations are high and my OCD is in overdrive. He's doing a great job, but I need more tweaks. I send him back to the drawing board for another edit.

I need to do everything right.

Margaret and Patrick head to the hotel where we've blocked off rooms for family. I decide this is a great time to catch up on my journaling. I'm working only a short time when I hear someone at the front door. It's a sweet lady I know from the retiree coffee klatch who lost her husband two years ago and has been grieving hard ever since. She sent me beautiful roses earlier in the day and is now delivering a dozen subs from Jersey Mike's.

I remember when Dave and I went to her husband's memorial. I cried far more than would be expected, being that her husband was not a close friend of mine. When we left, I told Dave all I could think of was that someday I'd be watching *my* Dave's memorial. All he said was, "I figured that's why you were crying so much."

This poor lady tells me that she's been sleeping on the couch for two years because all she can see in her bed is the last image of her husband violently coughing with COVID. I think of how differently we all process grief. The first thing I did was crawl into my bed, on Dave's side, and wrap myself in the bright-blue sheet and the yellow pillow that last touched his body.

Wednesday, November 1

Today is another day of planning. Tracey has done an amazing job handling food for Friday after the cemetery and Saturday after the memorial service. We're expecting about forty people, all of whom are family and close friends. I'm so glad I asked her to take care of this; I knew she was the perfect person for the job.

This afternoon my BFF from New Jersey and her husband are flying in for the weekend. As much as I'm looking forward to seeing all the family that's coming, all of them were Dave's people before we married and became *our* people after we married. Our friends from Jersey were *my* people before I knew Dave, so there's something particularly comforting about knowing she will be here soon.

While talking to her and her husband, I share for the first time all the details surrounding the last eight days of Dave's life: the days he never left the bed except to stand to relieve his bladder, the tremors, the hallucinations, all of it. These have been the worst days of my life, yet they're also intertwined with some of the sweetest and funniest memories of Dave.

By the time I'm ready for bed, I'm exhausted. As I go through my bathroom routine, I reach into a drawer for something. This drawer has always been used by Dave for extra deodorant and soap. Seeing his spare toiletries causes me to spin around to open the drawer in our vanity he used every day, the one with the razor, shaving cream, hairbrush, and deodorant. I look at the hairbrush with the loose gray hairs and fan my thumb through the bristles, somehow stunned that those hairs were once on his head. I open his deodorant and put it to my nose. Mmmm . . . smells like Dave. Sitting on the edge of the tub, I close my eyes while holding the open deodorant he used to swipe on his armpits every day. I love that smell. I miss that smell.

Thursday, November 2

*T*he earlier part of today is not too demanding; the only funeral-related chore I have to complete is the final revision of the memorial video. I've been an absolute pain in the ass to Nora's husband who has been working to make this perfect for me. I even apologized to Nora for putting so much pressure on him. Well, it's done now and he did a terrific job! The video shows the best of the best memories of Dave.

As I review the lineup for the memorial service, I suddenly see I may have a glitch. First the video with music plays, then Bobby speaks, followed by four other speakers. The music is picked out. Of course the version of "Somewhere Over the Rainbow" that Dave and I loved will be played during the service. Megan told her father months ago that she wanted to speak at his funeral. I realized when looking at the lineup that I'd put her right at the beginning, after the video.

She's on her way up from Florida at the moment, so I texted her to ask whether she thinks she'll be able to compose herself after the video quickly enough to speak or if she'd like me to change the order. She said, "If I'm terrible, people will forget." She has her father's sense of humor. She'll be amazing! I know the gist of what her words will be, and they're absolutely perfect.

Other than finalizing the video, things are quiet. Family have started checking into their hotels and are dropping by our . . . my . . . house. They started popping in to say hello around 3 p.m. Being an only child who comes from a very small family, I'm not used to having a lot of people around. And not just people, but family, which is different from people. Family interacts differently than friends; there's this unspoken acceptance of who you are and what you do. I actually find it all quite odd, and it's taken me years to get used to being part of a large family since I married Dave.

Dave's three siblings are here, and each of them came with their spouses, along with three of our grandsons, two nieces, and three of their daughters. They really are a beautiful family, with all the normal quirks, compassion, and love. I wasn't born into a family like that, so I consider myself pretty lucky to have married into it.

I look around the room. Other than the children, most of these people have known Dave longer than I have. Dave and I were married for twenty-one years and together for twenty-two and a half. They all have so much more history with him. I love hearing their stories and wish I'd been a part of those earlier days. I wish I'd known Dave back when he was a young man, even though I know with me being eleven years younger than he was, that wouldn't have been possible.

I feel guilty that I didn't realize what a gem Dave was when I first married him. People loved Dave, even his employees. He exuded kindness to everyone whose life he touched. Of course I loved Dave when I married him, and I knew he was a kind, humble soul. After all, I did chat with him for seven years before ever agreeing to go to Hawaii. But even throughout our first thirteen years of marriage, before we retired, I don't think I really understood how good a person he was. I'm feeling guilty now that I didn't love him harder the first thirteen years of our marriage, that I didn't give him what he deserved. I certainly didn't know how much he loved me at the time or how that love would change my life.

The eight years following our retirement included a five-month separation, a realization we wanted to make our marriage work, some therapy work, then a three-year cancer journey. We grew together more during those last years than some do after fifty years of marriage.

With all this company, my sisters-in-law have taken control of the kitchen, which I've relinquished completely for the first time in my life, and they're providing a steady supply of food and drinks. There is no need for me to assume the role of hostess.

My eyes wander around the room at all these mini-groups of people having conversations, and all I can think of is that Dave should be here. Every other time I've been to one of these family gatherings, Dave was here. He should be here. And why is he the first to die? I really do love these people, and I wouldn't want anything to happen to any of them, but why is my Dave the first to die? Dave is probably a better person than I because he never would have asked that question, much like the way he never asked, "Why me?" when it came to cancer. He certainly wondered why he got a rare cancer, as nearly nobody had heard of sinonasal cancer. But as far as getting cancer? He never asked, "Why me?"

The funeral is tomorrow, and the memorial is on Saturday. Dave and I talked about having the memorial on Saturday so more people could attend. I suppose under more traditional circumstances, the order would be to first go to the funeral home, followed by a service at the church, then a procession to the cemetery, then to the repast. However, we're having the events on two consecutive days, and family and close friends have traveled some pretty long distances. I don't see how I can send all these people back to their hotels after the memorial service, so I've invited those who were also at the funeral back to the house after the memorial as well. Now, I'm thinking having two gatherings at the house was a mistake. But it's too late to change anything. Dave would have thought it was a great idea to have two parties. What he didn't want was multiple viewings at the funeral home where people stood around and mourned. For that matter, there isn't any viewing. There will be very little time to stand around and mourn.

Tomorrow, before the funeral, I will see the open casket, just how we planned it. Then the funeral director will close the box and invite the rest of the family in to give them an opportunity to kneel at the casket and say a prayer. We will then journey to the cemetery in a procession and after that come back to the house.

I know that today's impromptu gathering was just a warm-up, and with less than half the people who are expected to arrive over the next two days. My company stayed for about five hours. I don't know how I'm going to do this for two days. I feel like I'm only partially present. It's like when Dave was having those episodes of one foot in one world and one foot in another. I just feel fuzzy.

I finally took Sadie out for a walk in the cold evening air, and I thought about how Dave was so better suited for this than I am. He would have made everyone comfortable, kept his grief to himself, and used humor to relieve any tension. I managed to hold it together for the most part. Well, I did until everyone left.

I still want that three-carrot ring to put in the box. It's been nagging at me that I haven't found it because it's impossible that I threw it out. I can't believe I didn't tear the house apart six months ago looking for it.

Well, tonight I found it. But in finding it I was absolutely devastated.

After all the company left tonight, Margaret, Claire, and I finished cleaning up the kitchen. They're both staying with me for several more days, thank God. I said goodnight and headed to my room to get my funeral clothes ready. While standing in my closet, I looked up to the shelf right over where *the* dress is hanging and noticed the straw box, the one Dave and I were gifted when we went to Hawaii on our very first trip, the trip where Dave was a perfect gentleman and slept on the balcony all week. Every night when we returned to our room after dinner, we had gifts waiting for us from the company hosting the trip. The straw box was one of those gifts. I instantly remembered this had been my keep-it box for stuff that Dave had given me. I opened up the box, and right in front of me was the three-carrot ring.

I'm thrilled that the ring turned up, but I saw all the beautiful and funny notes and letters from Dave from the early days . . . all the name tags from our fancy trips . . . all the cards that came on flower deliveries to my workplace. I can't believe I didn't go through this box with Dave. How could I have forgotten about it? How could I have been so stupid? For months now I've thought of everything so I would have no regrets. Now, as I rifle through the box, the more I read, the harder I cry. "How could I forget the box?" I keep saying through tears over and over. How did I not remember to share this with him? When we went through my other keep-it box, how did I not realize there was nothing in it from Dave? It would have been so much fun to go through the box together.

Just looking at some of the notes he wrote, I really can't believe how much he loved me. I fucked this up. Why did I not go through the box with him? How did I forget? Now he'll never know. Now he'll never know I saved all these mementos, most of them from the first five years of our relationship. I'm such an idiot!

I stumble out into the living room where Margaret and Claire are sitting. I sob, sputter, and cry while explaining what's in this box, how I forgot to share it with Dave, and that now I will never get to. He would have been so happy to see the things I saved. I haven't looked in this box since before we moved eight years ago. I'm so upset with myself. I thought I said and did everything I needed to—no regrets—and now I have a regret and there's no fixing it.

I made a mistake. **My third mistake.** Damnit!

The only benefit to this is that now I have the three-carrot ring so I can put it in the box with Dave tomorrow, along with Buddy Bear and the coffee-shop hat. I suppose I would have been more devastated if I'd found the straw box a week from now and then couldn't put it in with Dave.

I'm so upset. I fucked up. I miss my Dave. I can't believe he's really gone. I don't know how I will get through the next two days. I'm really going to have to channel Dave. I don't know how I will get through the rest of my life. The tears are flowing freely now, and they just won't stop.

25

Friday, November 3

*T*oday is the day of the funeral. How does a woman even begin to mentally prepare for her husband's funeral?

I dreamt of Dave the second morning after he died. Oddly, I had another dream about him last night. It's a bit fuzzy, but in it I told Dave we needed to have more sex. I can just imagine the look on Dave's face if he were here and I told him about this dream. I don't know whether Dave is actually a spirit flying around me these days, but he would find that dream pretty funny and would probably say something like, "Well, I can make all your dreams come true." Yes, Dave . . . you certainly can.

Margaret and Claire drove me to the funeral home before anyone else got there. On the way, Margaret picked up two quarters lying in a collection of change in the console. She handed them to me and said, "Put these in Dave's pocket. Our brother always said to have fifty cents for the ferryman." I put the coins in my pocket and made a mental note of the four things I needed to put in Dave's casket.

Bart, the same man who did all the talking the night Dave's body was picked up, greeted me at the door. There was one person who arrived ahead of me: Pastor Bobby. I didn't ask him to attend the services until the ceremony at the cemetery, but he was there anyway. It didn't really surprise me, considering he has always seemed to be in just the right place at just the right time.

> *It's still dark when Dave and I enter the hospital to admit Dave for his surgery two years ago. We're still newbies at this hospital, are far from our home, and don't know our way around. We're novices on the cancer train and think this will be a one-and-done surgery.*
>
> *I eventually learn where the café is, every bathroom, the emergency room, the surgical waiting room, the library, the lab, the infusion center, and the chapel.*
>
> *Dave and I wind our way through the halls, me chatty with nerves, and suddenly we see Pastor Bobby. We're both surprised and relieved to see a friendly face. The hospital is nearly three hours from our home, but Bobby was "in the area." We talk and pray and he leaves us. Every time after that, when Dave and I walk down that hall and come around that corner, we—usually I—say, "That's where Bobby was standing that morning!" Dave would nod his head.*

Bart asks if I'm ready to go into the room. Loaded question. He offers to bring me a chair to set near the casket. "No, I'll stand," I tell him.

I'm pulsing with nervous energy. I carry only the small bag of items I will be placing in Dave's casket. Bart escorts me into the room.

The first thing I see is the United States flag draped across the casket. Dave served his country well as part of the Strategic Air Command in the United States Air Force from 1970–1974 at the bottom of a missile silo in Missouri. He used to always get a laugh when talking about where he served. He would say, "I was protecting civilization from communism . . . There I was in

the Macon Delta, Charlie to the left of me, Charlie to the right
. . ." Of course, he was clowning around; he had the utmost
respect for the young men who served in Vietnam. He actually wasn't accepting of the title "Vietnam Veteran" because
he felt it was stolen valor since he never left the safety of the
United States. I suppose "Vietnam-era Veteran" would have
been more to his liking.

I realize Bart doesn't want to leave until he knows the body
has been prepared to my satisfaction. I tell him it's fine. I want
him to leave me alone. I need to have this private viewing.
Dave knew I needed it. It's more than the fact that my dad had
a closed casket; I need to make sure Dave is really there and
that everything is done right. I made those two mistakes in the
beginning; first, when I wasn't persistent enough about diag-
nosing why Dave had a chronic bloody nose, and second, when
I let that same doctor go in and do the first surgery after cancer
was detected. I know his cancer wasn't my fault, but like I said,
that would be my last mistake regarding his care. And it was. I
was on point with everything else, and I'm not done.

A flood of tears ensues. This is not my Dave. This is a body.
He is wearing all the clothing I picked out, and he looks similar to my Dave, but how could my husband look so different?
I think back to the last twenty-four hours of his life and the
metamorphosis that occurred, and I see its effects on Dave.
His forehead is perfectly smooth and free of wrinkles; I'm still
dumbfounded that someone who could have had such a deep
furrow in his brow for over twenty years could lose that crease
within days of his death. His nose hole is cleaned out perfectly. Dave would never have been able to get it that clean due
to the pain and bleeding that would occur during his daily nose
maintenance. My poor guy. When I realize how much his tissue had deteriorated, I wonder how on earth he walked around
and functioned. He really was a BEAST. His love for his family
and his worry for me and his daughter kept him going.

Dave's mouth is a tight line. He never had a really full upper lip, and as the tumor grew outside of his nose hole, the skin where a mustache would be swelled. This caused his lip to turn under, just on the right side. Dave's lips remind me of an old lady who has smoked for more years than she should have and ended up with dozens of tiny little lines surrounding her lips. I am so focused on the tight line that is Dave's lips, it doesn't immediately occur to me that the tumor is no longer visible. Holy cow! The tumor is gone. The tissue is smooth and without the varying shades of redness it had for months.

Much like during the last eight days of our lives together, I can't keep my hands off Dave. He is cold, but his skin still resembles the feel of skin. I touch his forehead and his cheeks. I play with his ears. He loved when I would rub and tug on his ears, much like the dog does.

He still has the same soft stubble on his face. I'd assumed the person who prepared Dave's body would shave his face. Dave liked to be clean-shaven, and I'm a touch annoyed with myself for not clarifying this detail. His skin was always so soft and smooth when he was freshly shaved. I think of that day he leaned up against the bathroom vanity, me sitting on the stool behind him holding him, and he asked, "You think I should shave?" I think about how during the last eight days his whiskers continued to grow and became softer as the days went on. My fingers were drawn to his squishy, furry chin when he was in our bed and unable to communicate with me, and they still are.

I run my hand down his hairy arms. His arms still look like Dave's arms. Thinner, but I always said he had "Popeye forearms." Strong and manly. These are the arms that have comforted me hundreds of times over the years. These are the arms that have pulled me close after my nightmares when Dave was playing the role of the big spoon lying in bed.

His hands are gently laid across his sunken belly. I think back to Sunday night when I was able to cradle my head on his belly while I listened to "Somewhere Over the Rainbow."

With tears flowing constantly, I toss the used tissues into the bag I brought. I pull Buddy Bear out of the bag, fix his Christmas ribbon, and tell him he has a very important job to do: I can no longer watch over Dave; he has to take on that job now. Eternally, this will be Buddy Bear's job. I place Buddy Bear near Dave's left shoulder.

I pull Dave's favorite bucket hat from the bag. A slideshow of memories flies through my mind of all the places Dave and I have been while he wore this hat. I place the hat above his right shoulder.

Next is the three-carrot ring, the ring that caused me so much grief last night. I'm glad I found it in the nick of time, but I'm still so disappointed that I hadn't found it sooner. It was months ago that I started thinking about the ring. If only I'd looked for it then, I would have eventually found the box with all the other mementos Dave gave me and we could have reminisced together.

I don't think Dave knew just how sentimental I can be. Maybe he did and he just liked to tease me about my lack of sentimentality. Unlike Dave, I have a reputation for being very practical. I'm the one who throws out Playbills and ticket stubs. Yet I have the Playbill from *Phantom of the Opera*, which we saw the night he asked me to marry him. I have to trust that as well as Dave knew me, he knew I had a sentimental side. At least I did when it came to him. But it still would have been so much fun to go through that box together . . .

I leave the plastic ring in its plastic box and gently place it under Dave's fingers. I suppose it's appropriate that a gag gift would make it into my husband's casket. He loved being funny!

The last item is the fifty cents for the ferryman. I take the quarters out of my pocket and tell Dave, "Tom says you may need these for the ferryman" as I slip them deep into the right pocket of his shorts so they don't fall out.

I glance at my watch and see that only five minutes have passed. I feel like I've been here for an eternity; how could it only be five minutes? I talk to Dave about how much I love him, how much I miss him, how much I feel I didn't appreciate him during the early years. I tell him that when I said I'd be okay and would have friends and family who'd care for me, I was lying. I didn't believe I would be okay then, and I don't believe it now.

I keep thinking, *This isn't Dave . . . this isn't Dave.* I finally look up at the ceiling instead of down at his body. I pray his soul exists somewhere. I pray I am able to feel it someday. I beg if he can hear me he give me a sign he's okay.

After another five minutes, I slide open the pocket door that leads to the hallway, where I see Bart has brought the kneeler I've requested. There will be many prayers today. I wander out to the lobby as family start flowing in. Bart had set up the ropes past the first door, so visitors are steered through the door I entered in and towards the guest book. I wait in the doorway and Pastor Bobby stands with me for a while. I feel like I'm greeting people at an event, standing at the door and hugging everyone who enters. Bobby reminds me these people are here for me too and I do not have to play hostess.

Colonel Tom appears. During the last month of Dave's life, I told Tom that Dave said he would like him to wear his uniform to the funeral. Dave thought it would be a real kick. When I first told Colonel Tom about this, I was surprised that he didn't jump at the idea but said he would have to think about it. He was concerned that since he still wore that uniform to many functions, he didn't want to be reminded of the funeral every time he put it on. I was somewhat disappointed at the time, but I thought, *WWDD* (what would Dave do). Dave would say, "If it makes Tom uncomfortable, don't push it. It's more important that he's comfortable."

I was about 95 percent sure the Colonel would wear his uniform. He did! He looks outstanding! So impressive! I don't know whether Dave ever saw Tom in his uniform, but Tom is crisp and pressed, and the number of gold-colored medals hanging from his chest would make even a civilian want to salute. I ask him if I can hug him. "Of course you can," he says. He asks if I'm surprised he wore the uniform. I tell him I'm somewhat surprised. But I'm not really. He would do anything for Dave.

For the next forty-five minutes, people talk, hug, cry, pray . . . comfort each other. Eventually I get a cue from Bart that it's almost time to leave. He gets everyone's attention and turns the room over to Pastor Bobby. Bobby does what he does best. He tries to comfort the people in that room with his words.

I ride to the cemetery with Dave's brother, along with his wife, Joan, and their daughter, Mary. Tom is truly broken over Dave's death, but he hides it well. Tom is also a former marine, and he spent some time at the nearby base over fifty years ago. We will come very close to that base on our way to the VA cemetery. This drive must be triggering memories for him of when he and Dave were just boys. Dave and I attended his and Joan's fiftieth wedding anniversary only months ago. That was where Dave first wore the blue shirt he's wearing today. Joan has been a part of the family since before she married Tom. They all lived near each other and were all friends when they were kids. I'm jealous they have that history. I wish I'd known Dave when he was a kid . . . a teenager . . . a young man. Dave and I shared many details of our childhoods over the years, but I've never had such a yearning to have been a part of his early days than I do right now.

Mary, our driver, is Dave's first niece as well as his god-daughter. All the nieces and nephews would agree that Uncle Dave was the best, funniest uncle that ever existed. Naturally, we are the lead car for the ten-minute drive to the cemetery. I'm still stunned that the hearse in front of us is holding my husband's body. When we arrive at the cemetery, I see two airmen from the United States Air Force who were sent to pay respects and fold the flag that's on Dave's casket. The government keeps things on a rigid schedule. With burials being at 10 a.m., noon, and 2 p.m. you have only thirty minutes to get in and get out. There's a paved area under a pavilion that appears to be exclusively for funerals. I thought we would be graveside.

Once we're all situated under the pavilion, Pastor Bobby says a few words, then one of the airmen plays taps on his bugle. I've been to a few police funerals, and that song always runs a chill up my spine. The airmen fold the flag with such incredible precision that even the former marines who are present are impressed. Colonel Tom marches over to the airman holding the flag. I'm still impressed by his decorated uniform. The young airman presents the flag to Colonel Tom and salutes. The Colonel brings the flag to me. I didn't know he was going to deliver the flag; I thought it would be one of the young airmen. He bends down and runs through a monologue, beginning with "On behalf of the president of the United States." He's fighting back tears. He's looking into my eyes, so I try to maintain dry eyes to make it easier for him. He places the flag in my arms and leaves.

Bart comes over to escort me out of the pavilion. This must be the cue to give others the signal to leave. I finally get to give Megan a hug. It's a long hug. She jokes that everyone is watching. When people start leaving, I walk over to the casket one last time. I now notice that it's gray. I couldn't remember whether Dave and I had picked the gray one or the blue one the day we sat at our dining table planning the funeral. Hmmm . . . the gray looks nice. I love you, Bumpy.

Mary drives me home, where Tracey has done a fabulous job setting out refreshments. Catering isn't her business, but she entertains so often at her house that she's well-qualified for this job. There's plenty of food and drink. The first thing I do is jump out of my butterfly dress since I have to wear it tomorrow. Plus, I was freezing outside at the funeral.

The day is . . . a success. People are talking, reminiscing, and sharing love. Dave would have loved to have been here. He would have loved to tell stories.

I manage to keep it together all day. Secretly I hope people will leave by 3 p.m., but some stragglers are still here and it's now 6 p.m. WWDD? Dave would have been okay with it. If Dave were here, I would have been okay with it too. With that being settled, I pour myself a shot of bourbon and grab a seat at the table.

After the crew of family leaves, my buddies Margaret and Claire help me package up food and clean up. The food was good, but there's a lot left over. I don't think we had as many guests as planned. We won't have to cook for weeks with the amount of food that's left.

I go to bed the same as always: bathroom routine, take a sleeping pill, position the pillows, sleep on an angle with my head on Dave's pillow . . . hold Sloth close.

26

Saturday, November 4

*T*oday is the day of the memorial service at the church. I wake up with a stomachache, which is pretty much the same as every other morning lately. I walk around the house taking deep breaths, dressed in the same butterfly dress I wore yesterday. For some reason, I feel more anxious today.

The memorial service is beautiful. It starts with a procession of the family walking into the church while "Because You Loved Me" by Celine Dion plays. I walk in with Dave's brother Tom, and we sit in the front row together, Patrick sitting to my right. I feel a new connection with Patrick. Only those who were in the bedroom with me and Dave for a week, the way Patrick and Margaret were, can truly understand what transpired and the unspoken connection that developed. The emotional highs and lows were intense, unforgiving, and exhausting. I think they call this "trauma bonding."

The service is wonderful. Of course I think so, but many people comment that it truly does Dave justice. The memorial video is painful to watch, but surprisingly I keep my tears inside while I watch it. Megan, Colonel Tom, and Jeremy prepared their own words and speak them beautifully. Margaret does a reading Dave and I liked that was in the blue pamphlet from hospice. When I read it to Dave weeks ago, he said, "I like that. You can have someone read that at the memorial."

"The Ship" by Henry Scott Holland
I am standing upon the seashore.
A ship at my side spreads her white sails to the
morning breeze
and starts for the blue ocean.
She is an object of beauty and strength.
I stand and watch her until at length she hangs
like a speck of white cloud
just where the sea and sky
come to mingle with each other.

Then someone at my side says: "There, she is gone!"

"Gone where?"

Gone from my sight. That is all.
She is just as large in mast and hull and spar
as she was when she left my side
and she is just as able to bear her load
of living freight to her destined port.
Her diminished size is in me, not in her.
And just at the moment when someone at my side says
"There, she is gone!"
there are other eyes watching her coming,
and other voices ready to take up the glad shout,
"Here she comes!"

And that is dying.[1]

Megan is the first speaker. I don't know how she keeps it together, but she does her dad proud. She's amazing when sharing how her dad was brilliant at creating words. The one she talks about at the service is "intestiny," a combination of "intestinal fortitude" and "integrity." When Megan was in high school, she played traveling soccer. Dave was the ultimate soccer dad, traveling to every game and carrying a huge banner he made with the word INTESTINY. Dave tackled the last three years of his life with amazing intestiny. He certainly instilled intestiny in Megan.

In the middle of the service, the long version of "Somewhere Over the Rainbow" plays. I love the lyrics of that song. The last time I heard it was nearly a week ago when I played it over and over while my head was cradled on Dave's belly after he died. Once again, I half hum, half mumble the words, knowing the tears are inevitable.

Pastor Bobby shares some words of hope and love, followed by Colonel Tom and Jeremy. These best friends of Dave both share some fun memories. I know they're both hurting badly over losing Dave, yet being such different people they handle it differently.

After the service, most of the family lines up across the front of the church, including me, Dave's children, and Dave's siblings. Dave and I had spoken about this type of "receiving line." He absolutely wanted this lineup because he wanted his friends to meet his brother and sisters. Dave spoke so often and proudly about his kids; I imagine most people felt like they knew them already. I have no idea how many people pass by offering hugs, kisses, and words of love and support. The entire experience is exhausting. I'm able to wear my survivor face for most of the procession. Only a couple of times I have difficulty holding back the tears.

All the family comes back to my house. Damn. Just saying "my house" instead of "our house" is a painful reminder Dave is no longer here. I feel like it took me so many years to say "we" and "our" and now I'm back to saying "I" and "mine." I don't like it. Anyway, the family comes back for an instant replay of the day before. There's food, drinking, stories, and some laughs. I keep chugging along because Dave would have loved it.

The high point is that two of Dave's air force buddies are here today. I've met Meyer before and thoroughly loved listening to him and Dave reliving their memories of the days when they were just boys serving their country in a cornfield in Missouri. But I also get to meet "Wags." I've heard so much about Wags over the years! He's certainly surprised when I ask him about the horse saddle he and Dave stored on the refrigerator of their apartment, something he didn't know I knew anything about. I sit and have lunch with Wags and his wife and share how Dave patiently reeled me in over seven years before I agreed to go out on a date. In exchange, Wags shares some of their crazy air force stories.

When all the family leave, they share hugs and words of support with me. However, they all leave with their spouses and have no idea how that felt for me. How could they? I share this thought with Margaret. She replies, "At some time in their lifetime, fifty percent of the people in that room will know just how it feels." She is right. Half of those spouses will someday become familiar with the grief of losing your person. I never thought of that before.

After everyone else leaves, Margaret, Claire, and I wrap up all the food, placing most of it in the freezer for meals to have weeks from now. Then we sit on the couch. This has been the nightly routine for days and is when organic conversations happen. I know they are here for me, not just for practical support but for emotional support, but I really don't know what they can do for me at this point. I can't even explain how I'm feeling.

For starters, I feel like a veil is covering my life. Everything seems just a bit cloudy. It's almost like having a sinus headache and feeling pressure in my head. I feel like that most of the time. I generally don't sit and think about Dave. I can't bear the thought. I've always had such a difficult time with the concept of death. I wonder whether anyone else in the world is like me. I also can't understand why I feel so surprised by his death. Surprised isn't even the right word because his death was expected; we planned it for weeks and made all the preparations. My role as Dave's loving wife and caregiver shifted from keeping him alive and happy to seeing him through a painless, quiet death. I know that was my role, so why does it feel so overwhelming and confusing now?

Sunday, November 5

I wake at 4:30 a.m., pleased that I slept through most of the night again. Sheer exhaustion (and sleeping pills) have assisted me in getting some quality sleep. But I start thinking about the incredulity of Dave not coming back. He's really gone! He's really gone forever!

I toss and turn for hours, knowing I need to get up at a respectable hour because we're having company for coffee before some of our family make the journey home. I'm glad we turned the clocks back last night, as I'm sure we can all use an extra hour of sleep.

Finally, our company comes and goes. I've pictured this time for months, the time when most everyone leaves and all the hubbub is over. Margaret and Claire will stay on for a few days. Margaret will return first, and Claire has offered to stay on as long as I need. She can work virtually and swears this isn't an inconvenience. It's always an inconvenience to stay in someone else's home, but I'll ask her to stay until I get the will and the life insurance sorted out. After that, I think I just want to be alone. Truth be told, I just want to mope around and feel sorry for myself, and I have a difficult time doing that in front of someone else.

A couple of years after Dave and I were married, we saw the movie *Shall We Dance*. We both enjoyed the movie, but I absolutely loved it! There's a line that Susan Sarandon's character says at a time when she thinks her husband might be cheating on her. She's hired a private investigator to find the truth and says to him, "We need a witness to our lives. There's a billion people on the planet . . . I mean, what does any one life really mean? But in a marriage, you're promising to care about everything. The good things, the bad things, the terrible things, the mundane things . . . all of it, all of the time, every day. You're saying 'Your life will not go unnoticed because I will notice it. Your life will not go unwitnessed because I will be your witness.'"[2] There were many things I loved about this movie, but those last couple of lines . . . boy, they stuck with me. Maybe my being an only child and having a lonely childhood has something to do with it.

What I never realized until the end of Dave's life was that I'd need a witness to the precious moments I spent with him. I was *his* witness until the end of his life, but what about me? Who would be *my* witness during those life-changing moments at the end? If it weren't for Margaret and Patrick, I would have been the only one. So, during dinner with Margaret and Claire tonight, I ask Margaret to share with me what she witnessed. Her words affect me so deeply that I ask her to write them down:

When Dave was in pain, it was Patty's touch that comforted him. When anxious, it was the sound of her voice that brought him calm. When he grew agitated, he was soothed by her embrace. The weaker Dave became, the stronger Patty grew. It was like watching the ebb and flow of the ocean on a beach. Dave was able to move away from the "now" into "the mystery of the next" because Patty was beside him, comforting him with her touch, calming him with her voice, and soothing him through her embrace. Her ability to let him go while also holding him secure remains for me a source of awe, humility, and gratitude. What his son Patrick and I were blessed to bear witness to those days was far more than love.

I can't figure out why I find it so important that someone else was able to witness Dave and me during the last few days of his life, but I just know that it is.

After dinner, Margaret and Claire go for a walk, and it's the first time I have the house to myself in weeks. I cry harder than I ever have in my life. I believe it's called "ugly crying." I shout, I curse, I beg. I wish I could believe Dave's soul is still around. I wish I could believe he is still here watching over me. But truthfully, I think that's crap. I think the end is the end and that's all there is. No Heaven, no golden gate, no floating around able to see your Earth-bound loved ones. As I said to Margaret, clear and convincing evidence is going to be hard to come by. But I won't believe in something just to make me feel better. That seems so childish.

When I was four years old, my mother flushed my turtle down the toilet. She told me he was getting too big for his bowl and was going to the ocean. The truth of the matter is, she had set his bowl on a radiator because our apartment was cold. She thought she was keeping him warm, but the poor turtle cooked on the hot radiator during the night. That may be a fine story for a four-year-old, but it wouldn't work now. And to believe that Dave is a spirit watching over me just to make me feel better seems absurd. The only truth is that Dave is no longer in pain. And that is a significant truth.

It's just over six weeks ago. Dave wakes up and swings his feet to the floor like he's done thousands of times before. This time when he puts pressure on the ball of his foot, he feels intense pain. I'm standing right there with his robe and slippers when I see the look on his face. For some reason, his foot cramps up. I firmly massage it, trying to relieve some of the tightness. It helps enough for him to be able to stand.

That afternoon, I suggest to Dave that I give him a foot rub to continue to ease the tightness in the ball of his foot. Dave sits in the pink chair facing me as I sit on our sofa. I use some cream to massage his feet slowly and deeply. As I rub, I speak.

"Dave, you know how I am at that moment of death with the dogs? That split second where they're alive" . . . I tilt my head to the left . . . "Dead" . . . I tilt my head to the right . . . "here" . . . tilt to the left . . . "not here" . . . tilt to the right.

With that, Dave says, "In pain . . . no pain."

Four days before Dave died, Chris-from-the-beach sent me a text saying, "Seven weeks down, thirteen hundred more to go." She was referring to the fact that her husband had passed seven weeks prior and, assuming a normal life span, she would live another twenty-five years, about 1,300 weeks. At the time I read it, I thought how morose it was. Of course I didn't say that to her, though. I realized she was in a dark place, and I tried to offer some words of encouragement, but no one could really help. Now I know why she said that. I feel exactly the same hopelessness, and I'm only in week one. I can't even fathom that this will continue to get worse before it gets better, and I can't begin to see how it will get better. I have so many feelings coming from different directions and I don't know how to cope with them.

Tomorrow I will see Mandy, the psychologist I've been seeing for about eight years, on average once a month. Often, times are quiet, but I continue to see her just to keep her posted on my life and keep my OCD in check. I never think of my OCD as being problematic; actually, I never think of it at all. Mandy first met Dave when she helped us after our temporary separation. She helped me get through a crisis I was going through at that time. I'm going to increase the frequency of my visits with her to once a week. I can foresee slipping into a depression. Dave would be so upset if he were to see that I let my life deteriorate. Then cancer will have taken two lives.

It's now exactly 3:25 p.m. One week ago this minute, Dave was still breathing. I knew he wasn't going to stay long in this world, but he was still here. Then it occurs to me we changed the clocks back last night for daylight savings time, so it's really 4:25 p.m. He's already been gone for just over one week.

Monday, November 6

*N*ow that the family has returned home, except for Margaret and Claire, I need to get down to business. I made a mental list last night of tasks I need to do and put some reminders in my phone. I set the bar low, with a goal of getting only one thing done each day. Last night I started writing thank you cards. I'm embarrassed to say I hate writing thank you cards. That would have been Dave's job . . . if he were still here. He had a way with words.

I've been piling things on my dresser for the last week and finally sorted through some of it. I looked in the bag that Pastor Bobby packed up after the memorial, which had the guest book and the memorial cards inside. I saw there were three out of four boxes left. That means I still have around 225 out of 300 cards. How could that be? I started counting signatures in the book and noticed most of the family signed in at the funeral as well as at the memorial. So that means, not including family, there were only about thirty-five friends at the memorial? That's impossible! There had to be at least a hundred people there.

I started sending some messages to friends, asking them where the book was placed at the service. It seems some people may have come in a different entrance. I don't really care about people not signing the book, but I want everyone to have a memorial card. I know anyone who ever met Dave could never forget him, but it's incredibly important to me that everyone has something tangible to show he existed. It's just my own quirkiness about death.

I still need to do everything right.

I decided to slip a couple of memorial cards into the envelopes with the thank you cards, especially for people who couldn't attend either of the services. I also wanted to send memorial cards to the most important members of our team at the university hospital, so I pulled out three envelopes and grabbed three memorial cards and three bright-blue sticky notes. On the sticky notes, I wrote "Remember him!" I know they will anyway. Even with hundreds and hundreds of future patients, I know they will remember Dave and me.

I know Dr. Thorn's address by heart. He was in a separate building off the main campus of the hospital. I addressed his envelope, slipped in the note and card, and sealed it. I wasn't sure whether I should use the hospital address for Mario and Dr. Shilo, so I attempted to send a quick message through the patient portal asking Mario for the address. I opened my Mac and clicked the ever-familiar icon. I knew Dave's username and password would populate automatically. It did. Then I got this message: "This account is inactive." Inactive. Dave is inactive. I sat there for a moment feeling like I'd been punched in the gut. Ultimately, I addressed the cards to be delivered to the hospital address.

My first task after that was to deal with banking issues and life insurance. I spent a couple of hours making phone calls. I called the investment guy for Dave's 401(k), emailed the life insurance guy, and contacted the probate office at the county. The probate clerk informed me there's a difference between filing a copy of the will and probating the will. I called the social security office because the information I needed isn't available on their website. The recording told me I would have a hold time of one hour and eighteen minutes. I decided to pop in my ear pods and start doing chores while remaining on hold. Then I grabbed Sadie to walk her down the street for her morning walk. I took a pad and pen with me just in case a live person picked up the phone. After thirteen minutes, my call was disconnected. Figures.

I've had an orange slip of paper sitting on the counter since we came back from the funeral on Friday. Apparently the post office had tried to deliver something that required a signature. I wasn't sure whether they would attempt to deliver it again today or hold it at the post office, and it occurred to me that I could pull up an image of the envelope online using the USPS Informed Delivery service. When I pulled up the images and checked what the mail was for Friday, my stomach dropped. It was a certified letter from the Onslow County Board of Elections. I knew it couldn't be good and thought there had to be something wrong with Dave's absentee ballot. How could that be? Patrick proofread the document after I completed it, and we both signed that we witnessed what Dave's wishes were.

I needed to get out, so I told my sisters-in-law I was going to do some errands. As I headed to the coffee shop, I thought of the alleged signs I got from Dave the day after he died: the sloth-like turtle, the song at the coffee shop, and the loose dog. I was skeptical then. I'm still skeptical. I'm also still praying . . . begging . . . pleading for Dave to give me a sign he's okay.

As I pulled up to the coffee shop, I negotiated with myself: "If 'Somewhere Over the Rainbow' is playing when I get out of the car, I will believe it is a sign. If every time I get out of the car in their parking lot, I hear that song, then I would have to believe. That would be clear and convincing evidence."

I pulled up to my usual parking space and hopped out of the car. I grabbed Sadie from the back, as well as the container Ashley used for the chicken soup and a pie plate that held a taco pie from her mom. They were kind enough to deliver food to me last week. Some upbeat beachy tune was playing through the speaker. I pretended I wasn't disappointed, then went inside.

Last month, stopping at the coffee shop without Dave to pick up his daily pineapple–mango smoothie wasn't an emotional task because he was still alive. Now . . . it's different. I know it will be weeks before I can sit at "our table." Dave and I had a conversation about this very topic about six weeks ago.

We walk into the coffee shop with Sadie. The girls know our regular drinks and prepare them the minute they see us. As always, they manage to fix our drinks, and Sadie's pup cup, amid all the other customers. They slyly slip our cups onto the counter. Our names, "I love you," and "Dave is the man" are written on them. We slip past the line, Dave drops a five in the tip jar, and we grab our drinks to head for our table.

I've always chosen the last table by the exit door, so this has become "our table." I ask Dave if the situation were reversed and I was the one who was going to die first, would he find coming to the coffee shop painful because of the memory of me, or would he find it comforting because of the memory of me? Naturally, Dave knows why I'm asking this question. He says, "If I were sitting in the same seat and you had passed, I would imagine you sitting across from me, and that would provide me comfort."

Eventually, I will sit in the coffee shop with Sadie, but today is not that day. Ashley made my drink and a pup cup for Sadie, and we headed out the door.

When I arrived at the post office, I was glad to hear the letter was there. I grabbed it, mailed the thank you cards, and purchased more stamps. I have many more thank you cards to write. *Dave, this is your job.*

As soon as I got in my car, I opened the letter and saw the first line: "The ballot submitted by the above-referenced voter has been challenged pursuant to North Carolina General Statute." My eyes scrolled down to see the words beside the checkbox: "The person is dead." That's why Dave's absentee ballot is being challenged! Patrick and I completed this weeks ago; Dave was sitting right there. I actually read it out loud to him even though we'd discussed quite a bit about who we were voting for in this local election. Dave was very much alive when this ballot was mailed in. Now, Election Day is tomorrow. The letter informed me that the county board will conduct a hearing on November 17 at 11 a.m. at the county Board of Elections office. That's my birthday. So, on my birthday, I will perform my last job as Dave's advocate. Regardless of whether his preferred candidates win, I am appalled that his vote will not count.

When I arrived home, I burst through the door to tell Margaret and Claire about this stupid letter. While Margaret searched the statute on the computer, I called the Board of Elections office. I learned that in North Carolina the law states that early voting is considered to be an extension of Election Day, so all the conditions that apply on Election Day need to be applied to early voting. One of those conditions is that to have a legal vote, a voter needs to be alive. Simple as that. If you're not alive on Election Day, your absentee ballot vote doesn't count. Son of a gun. Dave would be pissed. I am too.

I had about an hour to eat some lunch before I needed to head out to my 2 p.m. appointment with my therapist . . . my paid friend . . . Mandy. I haven't seen her since October 16, but I've been texting her to let her know what's going on. I really don't know where to start. I also don't know how she can help me.

I spent my hour telling Mandy about the last two weeks of Dave's life, mostly the last eight days, the days I feel most traumatized over. They're the same days I was so focused on taking care of my husband that I never really thought about the end game . . . that he would die. I knew this was hospice. I knew he would die. But in the day-to-day, I was so tuned into Dave's comfort and care that I didn't actually think about the fact he was dying. I just thought about how his symptoms changed. I needed to do everything right.

Basically, I was right; there was nothing Mandy could say to help me. She could only listen. But she did say three things that stuck with me.

First, she reminded me about when I'd made an appointment for Dave to visit with her. Since she had seen us together when we were working through some marriage difficulties, she agreed to see Dave after his diagnosis. She recalled it to be about a year after he was diagnosed. It was at a point when he was convinced we weren't ever going to be free of cancer and that he was going to die from it. Dave asked Mandy to look out for me. It's no surprise that my husband's one wish was for my care after he was gone. She told me she would honor Dave by caring for me.

The second thing she said was that she's heard grief is often considered a measure of the love you were unable to share with the person you lost. In essence, the more love you have for someone at the time of their death, the more grief you will have. This suggested to me that this grief road is going to be a long one.

The third thing she said was more of a personal compliment. She said if she's ever in a position where she has to show up for her person, she hopes she has half the stuff I am made of. I was truly flattered.

Tuesday, November 7

I'm continuing to spend the days performing all the practical tasks that are left for the loved one of someone who has passed. I've written more thank you cards, a task I still don't enjoy but am starting to get the hang of.

I decided to try my luck by calling Social Security again today. Lucky day—the wait time was only forty-seven minutes. I put the phone on speaker and floated around the house doing light chores. After thirty-six minutes, the rep from Social Security introduced herself. I asked her to take my phone number in the event we got disconnected. No, she could not do that. I gently set the phone on the desk, afraid if I accidentally hit the red disconnect button I'd have to start from scratch. I told her I had three reasons for my call. The first was to report the death of my husband, a social security recipient. Bart from the funeral home said they would handle this task, and according to the gal I'm speaking to, they have. My second purpose was to file for the $255 one-time death benefit. I discovered this little detail over a year ago when I was researching if I'd be eligible to collect Dave's social security after he passed.

That brings me to the third reason for my call. When I called last year, I learned that I won't be able to collect the spousal benefit until I turn sixty years old. This was one of the issues Dave and I discussed when figuring out financial matters. If Dave passed before I turned sixty, the household income would drop by nearly a third. Once I turned sixty, I could file for the spousal benefit. I asked the rep about that and she told me I was correct. She also said I should call them in August 2024 to make an appointment to file the claim.

I haven't received a response from the life insurance guy I emailed yesterday, but I'm considering the fact he may be on vacation. I called the 800 number, and the bot welcomed me, then offered options for directing my call. I was somewhat shocked that the first option was, "If you are calling to report the death of an insured." I thought that option would be buried down around number four or five. I pressed 1 and spoke to someone with a thick accent. She asked questions that I struggled to answer, only because of the crackle in the phone connection. The call sounded as if it were going halfway around the globe, but her thick accent didn't help either. I took notes as she spoke, knowing my ability to retain anything is not ideal right now.

I also spoke with Dennis, the investment guy, yesterday. He was surprisingly compassionate for a money guy, and I wondered just how much Dave had spoken to him. He said he would be sending me an email and I could reply and attach a scanned copy of the death certificate.

Wednesday, November 8

Margaret packed the last of her clothes and toiletries today. I told her and Claire yesterday that I don't know how they can help me. I know they have lives to get back to, including cats, an ongoing house project, and jobs. Margaret has been here for about two weeks now, and Dave would want me to send her home. I asked Claire if she could stay a little longer. I don't know why, but I'd hate to send her home and then regret it.

When I called Sadie for her morning walk, I noticed the temperature outside was 66°F with a real feel of 71. Perfect November weather! We walked the beach instead of the street, so I tied a long-sleeved T-shirt (advertising my favorite coffee shop) around my waist in case it was windier near the ocean. It was absolutely perfect. No one was on the beach except the fishermen. In the distance, the shrimp trawlers were making their way back to shore with their nets strewn behind them and a flock of seagulls hovering to try to catch random shrimp.

I never imagined I'd retire to such a beautiful place. Actually, when I was a young, single woman, I never imagined owning a place by the beach. Dave knew it was always a dream of mine, so we made that dream come true when we bought our little beach condo five years after we married. Although he was never much of a beachgoer, he seemed to truly discover the beauty of coastal living, spending weekends at the Jersey shore. So I suppose it wasn't much of a stretch that we might consider spending the rest of our lives at the beach. I knew from the day I took my job in 1990 that I would be retiring in August 2015, and that's what I told Dave very early in our relationship. It would be a bit early for him to retire, but he was game.

Still, we had no idea where we wanted to move and didn't give it any thought. So it was no surprise when I told Dave in 2012 that we needed to start the process of finding our happy place. Being a perpetual planner and fueled by OCD, I figured two years would be enough time for planning. We knew we wanted to leave New Jersey, mostly because of the climate. We discussed the idea of moving south of Virginia, and after minimal discussion, we decided we wanted to live north of Georgia. That left North and South Carolina. The plan was to discover the coast of South Carolina in 2012 and North Carolina in 2013.

South Carolina doesn't pan out too well. It's actually one of our worst vacations ever, with neither one of us knowing exactly what we're looking for. Most folks spend their lives vacationing at a beloved place and know that's exactly where they want to move when they retire. That isn't us. So, the following year, I do a lot of research on the beach communities of North Carolina in the vicinity of Wilmington.

I rent us an Airbnb where we can stay over the four-day Thanksgiving weekend while we visit Wrightsville, Carolina, and Kure beaches. They are all lovely, but I can't find what I'm looking for, that je ne sais quoi. Dave lives by the philosophy, "Happy wife, happy life," so he will be content wherever I am happy.

I feel somewhat defeated and concerned that I don't know what our next step will be. We take a drive out of town one day, and Dave notices a highway sign that reads, "Topsail Island 22." How could I have missed this beach? We drive the twenty-two miles to the island. It's a beautiful day, complete with blue skies and low humidity. We cross a little swing bridge and drive north up the ocean side. The ocean isn't in view from the street, so we park, grab the two dogs, and head over the dune on one of the crossovers to the beach. The beach is big and wide, and the day is gorgeous.

We walk along the beach, watching the dogs run near the waves. After a fifteen-minute walk, I say to Dave, "I think this is it." I imagine he's incredibly relieved, and he tells me he likes it too. That's all it takes . . . just a feeling I have.

Naturally, Patty being Patty, I research the heck out of the area when we return home. Ultimately, we select one of the three municipalities that occupy the twenty-six-mile island, and I begin visiting regularly to look for a house for us. By November 2014, we purchase our beautiful beach house, a house I describe to Dave as "perfect just the way it is." I then continue to paint, rebuild, and change nearly everything in the house, something Dave teases me about for the rest of his life.

Today's weather was just like Thanksgiving 2013, and I thought back to that walk on the beach when I'd believed

I found our future happy place. Everything is different now, right down to the dog.

I rolled Dave's wedding band through my fingers. It's still on the chain around my neck. I thought about how Dave said I needed to get a stronger chain. I'm still torn about whether I want sterling silver, yellow gold, or white gold. How will I ever make all these little, commonplace decisions alone, especially those that turn into mountains for me? I'm great with major decisions, but not these. As I ran the ring back and forth on the chain, I whispered, "Please, Dave, let me know you're okay . . . please knock me over the head with a sign . . . I'm losing faith that you're still here."

People have very personal beliefs as to what happens when a person dies. Although the book I'm reading details inspiring and enlightening accounts of those brought back from near death, I am not convinced. I believe they're implying that if you die and aren't resuscitated, you'll continue through the tunnel to the bright light that offers comfort, love, and acceptance, and your spirit will exist forever in this alternate place. I do believe these documented accounts of people's experiences to be truthful and accurate, but I'm leaning towards the idea that this experience is temporary and manufactured by the brain. We all know we haven't tapped into the vast capabilities of the brain. What if this beautiful afterlife lasts for three minutes, then the light goes out and it's over? Just over. Over-over. People who come back from a near-death experience never reach this part of the journey; people who do reach it are unable to be resuscitated. So, it remains a mystery. Naturally, it's easier and more comforting to believe that life continues in an alternate form, that there's everlasting life, something I've struggled to believe since I was a young girl.

As Sadie and I made our way home, I noticed my much-neglected garden and the empty bird feeder. I've always been the "nature nut" in the family, but a bit of me wore off on Dave and he loved listening to my tales of feeding birds, watching baby birds in our birdhouses, and volunteering with a local bird rescue. I filled the feeder and decided to pull out the hose to give the garden a drink. As I walked around the side of the house I rarely walk on, I saw the half-barrel planter with the hydrangea.

Soon after Dave and I return home from Jamaica, Easter is approaching. The holiday will be an opportunity to introduce Dave to my mother. My mom knows the story of my trips with Dave, and I came home from Jamaica telling her I thought I'd found the guy I was going to marry and that he happens to work around the corner from where she lives. Knowing she would meet him on Easter at my house, she leaves a note on Dave's car saying, "Patty loves flowers . . . bring her flowers."

Dave brings me three blue hydrangeas that day. How he knows I love blue hydrangeas I'll never know. Even my wedding bouquet is made up of blue hydrangeas! I plant all three plants in the garden, and one grows to be massive, spanning five feet by the time we move fourteen years later.

When we move, I take two sections of this gorgeous hydrangea and attempt to root them at our new home in North Carolina. The climate is dramatically different, but I'm able to keep one alive in a container.

When I looked at my shriveled-up hydrangea, I saw that it wasn't dead, just very thirsty. It's now pink due to the acidity of the soil. That's okay . . . it's still from the same plant Dave gave me over twenty-two years ago.

I pulled out the hose and watered the hydrangea, then made my way to the memory garden, where I've created stones with all my departed dog's names. Most have a few words that embody their personalities. I've always enjoyed looking at the stones with their names because it gives me a moment to remember all the days I enjoyed with my four-legged children.

As I fanned the hose from side to side, somehow the water caught a prism and created a rainbow when the hose was in just the right spot with the sun over my left shoulder. When I moved the hose, the rainbow disappeared. The rainbow made me think of "Somewhere Over the Rainbow," which then made me think of Dave, which in turn made me think of the time I asked him if I should get a memory stone for him to put in the garden. He thought it was a good idea.

28

Thursday, November 9

*T*his morning I started the day like I have for the last eleven days: Before I even open my eyes, I remember Dave is gone. The first week after he died, I slept like the dead—no pun intended. Realistically, prior to Dave dying, I was sleeping with one eye open for months and months and was severely exhausted. And now, although I'm extremely tired by 8 p.m., my sleep has been restless. I wake up at least four times a night, and I never feel rested.

When I finally wake and see daylight, I roll to my left so I can lie on the yellow pillow that was Dave's and wrap myself tighter in the bright-blue sheet I'm still sleeping with. One of these days I'll have to wash them. Every morning, I quietly say out loud the same words as I squeeze the yellow pillow: "Good morning, Dave, I miss you." No tears come, but the emptiness weighs heavy on my heart. I go into the bathroom to brush my teeth and do my morning routine. I have strong, vivid memories of Dave in this small space. Some are awful, yet I also have the memories of our long Tub Talks when I'd stare at Dave's face to burn his image into my brain. This morning I pulled out my darkest lipstick and wrote, "I Miss You" on Dave's side of the mirror.

As I went about the morning, I remembered a friend from California I hadn't yet told about Dave's death. I pulled up the funeral home website to scroll to Dave's picture so I could send her the link to his obituary. I was quite surprised that I had to scroll through twenty-four names to get to Dave's picture. Twenty-four souls have been sent to their final resting place, and from just this funeral home and only in the last eleven days. I suddenly had an awareness that twenty-four families are grieving just like I am. There are three funeral homes in my immediate area, which means there are about seventy-five families in my vicinity who are grieving just like me. This indicates a huge likelihood that on any given day when I go to the grocery store, the gas station, or the pharmacy, I'll have an encounter with a grieving person.

I started thinking about how I've been going into stores over the last week and a half and probably appearing intro-spective or maybe even self-absorbed. But actually, the weight of the grief feels like an anchor around my chest. I've always considered the saying that you don't know what someone is going through until you walk a mile in their shoes, but I've generally considered more common problems such as family stuff, finances, and job problems. I've never considered some-one I walk by and share a quick word with might have the same anchor of grief around their chest that I do now.

I told Claire I was heading out to run a few quick errands. As I backed out of the driveway with Sadie in the car, my first stop was the coffee shop for my drink and a pup cup. I spoke out loud to Dave, "Bumpy, you know I really need you to knock me over the head with a sign. Please, please, before you go on to the next phase of your journey, I have to know you're okay. I have to know. Even if I just see a napkin blow by my feet with a picture of a blue butterfly, I will know . . . or I might even be okay with a bluebird at our feeder since we never see bluebirds this close to the beach. I have to know you're okay."

I headed into the coffee shop with Sadie, and the barista gave me a warm smile as she grabbed my protein drink to make my special concoction. Just then, Jaiden came out of the kitchen.

"Jaiden! I didn't know you were here," I said.

"I'm here," she replied as she jogged around the counter to give hugs to me and pets to Sadie. She gave me one of the tightest hugs I've felt in days. She's only seventeen years old, but she's so grown up. Dave adored her! As she fed Sadie her pup cup, she asked me how I'm holding up and inquired whether I've done any baking lately. I told her I haven't but I'm considering making my sweet potato muffins with dark chocolate chips. She crinkled her nose a little bit, saying she doesn't love sweet potatoes, but she offered to come over and help me bake. She loves to bake.

We said our goodbyes, and I walked into the next room where the tables are. Right before I got to the exit, I stopped at "our table." I remembered how Dave said if the situation were reversed, he would be comforted by sitting at that table visualizing me. I paused, stared at his chair, and saw his image. A lump in my throat formed immediately. *Not yet*, I thought. *I can't do this yet.* I opened the door and headed to the car with wet eyes.

As I drove across the bridge to leave the island, I made three quick stops. It was a beautiful breezy day, so I left the car windows open for Sadie. As I headed back to the island, I slowed down as I approached the roundabout prior to the bridge that crosses the Intracoastal Waterway. Just to my right were the half dozen single-wide trailers that have popped up in the last five years or so. There was a sign that caught my eye, one of those signs politicians print or a painter or landscaper uses to advertise their services. On the sign was a picture of a beautiful blue butterfly. I blinked my eyes and it was still there. I kept making right turns until I pulled up to the trailer with the sign out front. As I walked across private property and around to the sign so I could take a picture, a man came out of the trailer asking, "Can I help you?"

I stuttered and stammered, saying, "That sign . . . the one with the butterfly . . . where did you get it?" As he started to speak, I cut him off. I didn't really care where he'd bought it. "When did you put it out there?" I asked. He said about two weeks ago.

I'm sure I sounded a little crazy when I told him my husband died a week and a half ago and blue butterflies mean something to us. He told me the sign had been purchased in support of a little girl who's trying to get a kidney transplant and he could find out where to get another one if I wanted it. I told him I'd think about it, thanked him for his time, and walked around to take a picture. On this beautiful picture of the blue butterfly were the words, "Pray for Insley."

Is this my sign? I don't remember seeing it before. Maybe I did see it before. I think maybe I might have. Or maybe not.

When I got home, I told Claire the story and showed her the picture of the sign. "Oh my God, Patty," she exclaimed. "This is your sign!" She grabbed my shoulders and shook me as her eyes became as wide as saucers. "You can't deny this is your sign," she said. I smirked, suggesting it may be.

Dave knows me one hundred times better than anyone on this planet. If he is out there, he will find a way to convince me. The one and only thing Dave would want is to give me peace. He will find a way . . . if he can.

29

Saturday, November 11

I am overwhelmed with sadness today. Claire is here
with me for a few more days. Besides being extremely
sensitive, she's an excellent conversationalist and extremely
well-versed in just about everything. She's also a distraction.
Based on that description, I'm almost describing Dave, but
she's not Dave.

I spent the morning cooking chicken and rice for Sadie in
the instant pot. Sadie has been sick for a few days, and I'm
hoping she just ate something indescribable from the house
next door that's under construction. Then I baked chocolate
banana oatmeal for Claire and me. One time when I made this,
one of my grandsons said it looked like I was eating a brownie
for breakfast. I told him it was oatmeal. He insisted it looked
like a brownie . . . Nana is eating a brownie for breakfast.
Chuckle.

Dave was right that I need a stronger chain to hold his
wedding band around my neck. Today Claire and I drove to
the jewelry store that Dave and I used to frequent. I told my
sales lady, "I need a chain for my husband's wedding band. He
passed away two weeks ago." She offered her condolences and
we started sorting through chains. Sterling silver, yellow gold,
white gold, twenty-two inches, twenty-four inches . . . I'm
overwhelmed with decisions, as I knew I would be. Claire was
doing her best to offer advice. I kept thinking, *Why didn't I do*

this six months ago? Dave could have helped me. He's the only per-son who knows me inside and out. He's the only one who can help me resolve this internal conflict. It's just a chain for Christ's sake!

I have no idea how much time passed, but the sales lady remained patient; I give her credit for that. Essentially, she didn't know if I was going to buy the $80 silver one or the $3,200 gold one. Once I made a decision, I felt the emotion well up inside and my eyes begin to water. I was anxious to leave the store because it was getting harder to hold back the tears. Once in the car with Claire, I let them flow just a little. I never let loose completely when someone is around.

Claire offered to take me to lunch, so we stopped at Panera. As we waited for our food, I looked around the room at all the people. There were a couple of retirees similar to Dave and me, a young couple, a mom with two girls, and a few teenagers, all of whom seemed to be so carefree. Did any of them have the heavy heart that I feel right now? If so, how do they walk around faking it all day? And if they do fake it all day, do they crumble when they get home? Do they look upward and tell their loved ones how much they're missed, how they don't know how to go on without them, how everything seems so empty now? When the one you love dies and takes half your heart with him, you just feel empty.

When Dave was sick, I thought how someday, when he was no longer here, I would take the camper out on my own and do more camping. Not just traveling via RV like Dave and I did, but actual camping, including cooking outside and doing lots of hiking. That latter part wasn't Dave's cup of tea. In actual-ity, I don't even want to think about taking the camper out. All I can think of is that Dave was with me every time we pulled out of our driveway.

Will this feeling go away? Will the heaviness ever lighten? Will the memories of Dave and I traveling the country in the camper ever make me smile instead of making me feel sad and alone?

Claire picked up a $5 puzzle during our travels today. I haven't turned on the radio or the TV in nearly four weeks. I'm not quite sure why I'm isolating myself this way. Maybe I'm just trying to avoid triggers. The puzzle Claire bought is a scene of winter in New York City. This should keep us busy for a while. However, with my OCD tendencies, I usually become consumed with jigsaw puzzles, working on them for six, seven, even eight hours at a time.

As we were doing the puzzle, I got a text from Megan asking if I'll be coming to her house in Florida for Christmas. Several thoughts whizzed through my mind. The first was that Dave would have my head if I didn't spend Christmas with family. The second was that I don't know what I'm doing for Thanksgiving next week, let alone what I'm doing for Christmas. I put the second thought in a text and sent it to Megan. She didn't pressure me. She just wanted to let me know that James will be joining them again this year so she thought she would ask me too.

Last Christmas, Dave and I bring the camper down to Megan's house and park it in the driveway. Other than the fact that Florida is having an unusual cold snap, which presents a few temporary issues, this idea of camping in their driveway is the best of all worlds. We can visit with the kids when we want and have some space as well. James and his girlfriend stay at Megan's house for a few days.

One night, Dave and I are sitting in the camper watching a movie. Eventually we hear a little knock at the door. It's Teddy, Megan's middle son. Moments later, her youngest comes in. Moments after that, they're back and forth

*going from the camper to the house to pile all their favor-
ite blankets and pillows onto the twin beds we have in the
camper, each of them taking a bed. Soon after that, Megan
asks if we all want hot chocolate. The four of us sit in the
camper, Dave and me at the dinette and the kids in our
beds under piles of snuggly blankets, watching a Christmas movie and drinking hot chocolate. It was right out of
a Norman Rockwell scene. Since then, I remind Dave of
that night and what a special Christmas memory it is.*

Maybe it's the nostalgia of the Christmas question, but
suddenly I was focusing on the New York puzzle. Dave used
to take me to New York. He loved Broadway, the East Village,
Central Park . . . he loved it all!

I looked at the puzzle: *Phantom of the Opera*; we saw that the
night we got engaged. *Wicked*; Dave took me to see that too.
MetLife; Dave's life insurance is from there. Yellow taxis; they
remind me of a restaurant that had a taxicab theme and Mexi-
can food with great tortilla chips in baskets set on the tables.

*It's the year 2000. Dave and I have never been on a date.
It's before Hawaii and before we fell in love in Jamaica.
Dave tells me he has tickets to see* A Moon for the Mis-
begotten *on Broadway. I'm not sure why I agree to go,
but I do.*

*Dave picks me up at my house. I'm dressed in casual khaki
pants and a fitted black tank top. Dave later tells me that
this is the first time he saw me "looking like a girl" instead
of like a cop in uniform, and he's suitably impressed.*

*Dave drives us into New York City. He knows where he's
going, where to park, where to walk, and is very comfortable with his surroundings. I am not. I liked going to
the city when I was eighteen years old, and I enjoyed the*

nightlife, but I have long tired of the hustle and bustle and get a tad claustrophobic surrounded by all these people.

The show is fine. Personally, I prefer musicals to plays, but Dave doesn't know that about me yet.

We walk back to the car at around 10:30 p.m. At that hour and on a weekend, New York is just starting to pick up steam. The theater is on 48th Street between 7th and 8th Avenues. I have no comprehension of where we are or where we're going. I never relinquish control like this, but even on a first date, I trust Dave. As we're walking across a busy crosswalk back to the Marriott Marquis, Dave grabs my hand so I don't get separated from him. He just grabs it! My mind wanders to what he's thinking, but I don't really care. I feel safe. And, due to an experience I had when I was about seven years old with a boyfriend of my mother's, safe was a feeling I rarely felt with men. Trust was a feeling I felt with pretty much no one. Dave becomes the first person I learn to completely trust.

This mental walk down memory lane sent me into a tailspin. Moments later, I noticed poor Claire looking at me with my head in my hands, bawling my eyes out. Her compassionate nature helped me calm down, but I realized my grief is turning into more of a mental health issue than just routine grief. My OCD is causing me to obsessively run through the same thoughts over and over and over. I will see Mandy on Monday.

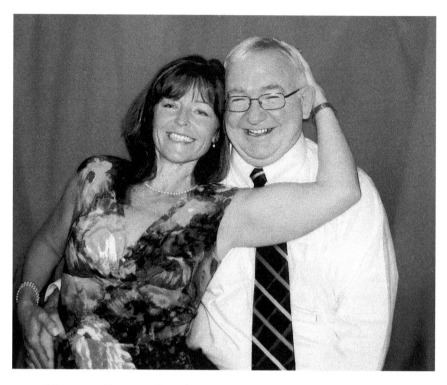

May 2011: Dave and me in a photo booth at a family wedding

30

Monday, November 13

*L*ast night I finished the book I've been reading about near-death experiences, or NDEs, and the concept of the soul/spirit/mind existing outside the body after physical death. This book was written in 1975, and I imagine there's a lot more current information on the subject now that nearly fifty years have passed. I'll consider doing more reading. I'm not sure whether these stories will provide me comfort, but I'll put the thought in my back pocket to pull it out at a later date if needed.

I had another restless night last night. My body tends to wake at 5 or 6 a.m., a time I used to rise, sit at the computer for a couple of hours, and drink my coffee . . . when Dave was still here. By the time he'd wake, Wonder Woman welcomed him into the day. But now I don't wake up as Wonder Woman; it takes me time to get there. Some days I never feel like Wonder Woman.

I fell back to sleep because I prefer to spend as many hours sleeping as possible. I used to fall into a deep sleep if I closed my eyes at an early morning hour. Now I fall into a state of dreamland. Last night I had a horrific nightmare.

> *I see Dave's face but just a sliver of the front. Dave is get-ting radiation treatment, but it looks more like a laser. They're blasting his cheek to kill the cancer. The laser*

resembles the kind you see in a cartoon or an action movie when the thief is cutting a hole in a safe with a blow torch. His face needs to have several blasts for just a few seconds each time. He grimaces, it's painful and burning him, but I beg him to withstand it a little longer. When the treatment is complete, I see his face. There are jagged holes burned clear through where his eyes and the apples of the cheeks should be. There's still no body, not even a head, just the front of his face. I suddenly realize he's dead, and I regret putting him through such discomfort when he was so close to dying.

I woke from the dream absolutely terrified! I've always been fairly adept at analyzing my dreams. My philosophy is to identify the emotion you were feeling in the dream. Most of the substance of the dream is irrelevant, just take the emotion. I felt guilty. Why would I feel so guilty? Guilty for not appreciating him in our early years together? I hope the picture of this in my brain fades.

If Dave were still alive, I would tell him I had a nightmare. He would ask me about it, and I would cry as I told him the dream. Then he would pull me close, letting me be the little spoon and he the big spoon while he'd whisper, "My poor Snookums."

After I poured my first cup of coffee, I climbed back into my warm bed to read more of the new book I started last night. Margaret gave it to me when she first came down to help with Dave. It's called *Signs* and is written by a medium. Margaret said to put it away until I was ready to read it. Being that this is an actual paperback and not an electronic book, I mark my stopping place with a hotel key card I found as I was rummaging through my nightstand for something that would serve as a bookmark. I've read a few chapters about the signs from the universe a person receives after the death of a loved one.

Instead of chalking up these unusual occurrences to coincidence, I'm supposed to be open-minded if I want to receive them.

When I was ready for my second cup of coffee, I grabbed the key card I used last night and slipped it into the book. I closed the book, then thought that the key card was upside down. My OCD was calling out to me, so I opened the book to make sure the key card was in the right-side-up direction. The words on the key card jumped out at me: "It's time to let me go." I never would have noticed if not for my OCD. I started to wonder whether this was a sign.

Later this morning, my phone rang and the name on the caller ID showed it was Dr. Shilo. Unlike when Dr. Thorn called, I wasn't positive it was Dr. Shilo, so I answered with a general hello.

"Patty, Stu Shilo here," he said.

"Hi Stu, I thought it might be you," I replied.

He was away last week and wanted to give me some time to myself. He was calling to see whether Dave and I got to share some quality time together. I had so much to share with him.

I told him about the last six weeks of Dave's life, about the first four weeks when Dave had a steady stream of visitors, and about how his appetite and energy increased at one point so we'd actually gone out to dinner. I talked about how awful the last two weeks were, how the first of those was awful for Dave and the latter was awful for me. I told him how Dave started to have tremors early on and that when I'd asked the nurse why, she explained it was his body transitioning. Dr. Shilo didn't seem surprised by this answer.

How did I not know this? The tremors continued over the next week or so, becoming quite severe, but only when Dave was awake. They didn't happen when he slept. Why isn't this in the blue book? Why doesn't anyone tell the caregiver of a hospice patient this will happen? Does anyone but hospice nurses know this happens to a failing body?

Dr. Shilo went on to say that Dave's resilience was remarkable and the care I gave to him was exceptional. When I asked him, he admitted he hadn't expected Dave to live as long as he did. We had often discussed in his office that we were in unchartered territory, not confined to the rigid barriers of protocols and trials. We were in a space where Dr. Shilo could try new things. Clearly that had paid off. I believe everyone involved, including Dave, didn't think Dave would live longer than a year after his first recurrence. Everyone except me.

I reminded Dr. Shilo that his office had referred us to palliative care for pain management only a week before our conversation with him, the conversation when Dave decided to stop all treatment. I explained that although I'm not looking to find fault, I believe palliative care should have been suggested many, many months earlier. Maybe even a year earlier! Prior to palliative care, Dave was taking such a strong painkiller that it put him to sleep, so he'd often opt to take less of the drug and be in more pain so that he could stay awake and enjoy his life. A person should not have to choose between those two options! It's possible that a low-dose fentanyl patch and some liquid morphine would have made a difference in Dave's quality of life by minimizing his uncontrollable pain.

Dr. Shilo agreed that there are many studies that show cancer patients benefit from early intervention of palliative care, but there's a cost. He said the medical community believes that when a doctor suggests palliative care, the patient believes the doctor considers them to be a lost cause and loses trust in the doctor. I can understand this to be true, as I remember when our team first suggested it to me less than two months before Dave's eventual death, I was completely disheartened by it. I also thought palliative care was the same thing as hospice, a seven-letter word for imminent death. It was Mario who had explained to me the benefits of early palliative care for pain management.

I started thinking about how when I updated our friends and family regarding Dave's care, I said, "We've enlisted the help of palliative care for pain management." I always intentionally added "pain management" to the update so people didn't think Dave was nearing the end of his life. I was afraid people would think we were giving up.

I think that's something we need to do better as a society. A cancer patient, or any other patient for that matter, should not have to choose between pain and quality of life. If palliative care can provide some pain relief, doctors need to feel confident when suggesting it that they will not lose the trust of their patients. We all need to understand that this is a quality-of-life medical service that is no different from when I consulted a dietitian, an acupuncturist, or the folks who perform hyperbaric oxygen therapy. Who's going to be responsible for educating people well before these services are needed? When are we going to start having these conversations instead of shying away from them?

Dr. Shilo said we are family. I always felt that way with him and Dr. Thorn. At the time, I wondered whether we were special to our medical team or if they had this type of relationship with all their patients and their families. I really believe Dave and I were, and still are, special to them.

*   *   *

My appointment with Mandy was at 1 p.m. today. Even though I'm quite proficient at using my online calendar, I have a terrible habit of forgetting when I factor in my travel time and when I don't, which often causes me to arrive an hour early. Today, I decided to leave an extra hour early because I was taking Claire with me so I could drop her off in downtown Wilmington and then we could grab lunch together after. Somehow in my head I ended up twisting the times and thinking I needed to leave at noon. I often used to confess to Dave my screwups in botching up appointment times, and he would just shake his head in disbelief. I'm so precise with everything else, but I often make this error.

As we headed out the door, Claire asked me when my appointment was. Looking at my calendar, I shouted, "Shit! Crap! I can't believe I did this again! How do I always do this?" Leaving at a few minutes to noon, the likelihood of me being able to drop off Claire and get to my appointment by 1 p.m. was slim to none. I considered all our options.

Not even ten minutes after we beat feet out of the house, I got a text from Mandy saying, "Hi Patty. I'm running about ten minutes late today." You're kidding. She has never texted me to tell me she's running late. A sign from Dave? Ten minutes was enough time to let me drop off Claire and still be timely for my appointment.

With Claire at her destination, I headed back in the other direction towards Mandy's office. On the way, I passed the restaurant that Dave, Megan, and I dined at the last time Megan visited. I looked up at the marquee-style sign and saw the words, "I'm crazy pho you." Another sign from Dave?

At this point, I was really anxious to get to my appointment with Mandy. My head has been all over the place dealing with grief, anxiety, OCD, and fear of the future, and now I wanted to tell Mandy about the signs I received today. I rambled on nonstop for at least half my session, my head feeling like a bubbling volcano and my OCD dominating me. I barely took a breath except to cry. But I did chuckle when I told Mandy about the signs. When I referenced her ten-minutes-late text, she playfully said, "So it was Dave who screwed up my day." What a beautiful thought!

Mandy finally gave me her thoughts. She thinks I'm not just dealing with grief but with trauma. She believes I've never taken the time over the last three years to process the trauma of Dave's cancer. All the ups and downs, the surgeries, the scans, the radiation, the chemo, the overnight visits to the out-of-town hospital, the constant anatomical changes, the never-ending dietary changes . . . the list goes on and on. I was so busy being in "fix-it mode," something I do very, very well, I never took the time to acknowledge the emotional impact of these changes. I was focused on being a cheerleader and a caregiver and did not consider how the cancer was affecting me.

Certainly plausible. There's nothing for me to fix now. Nothing for me to focus on. My brain is spinning trying to find something to do. It hasn't processed the trauma of the last three years, it hasn't even begun to process how awful the last two weeks of Dave's life were, and it's certainly unable to grasp the next twenty years.

Mandy suggested we spend some time dealing with this recent trauma. I knew she hit the nail on the head when I started crying. I always know I hit on a truth when I start crying in my therapist's office. She suggested that although it might not be ideal, my relationship with Dave may now consist of messages on bookmarks and restaurant signs. It's not perfect, but maybe that's what it is at this moment in time. I told her I've been overwhelmed with the feeling that I didn't appreciate Dave enough during our early years of marriage. She suggested I try to stay present and not dwell on the past or my fear of the future.

On the drive home with Claire, I turned the music on for the first time in nearly three weeks. "Ain't Nobody" by Chaka Khan came on from my playlist, a song Dave loved and used to bounce around to while sitting in his seat like a White boy feeling the rhythm. It always made me laugh.

It was only 5:30 p.m. when we arrived home, but it was dark already. Sadie was itching to go for a walk, so I took her out on the beach. As I passed the bench Dave and I used to sit on together, I took an extra-long glance at it, feeling his absence. I walked Sadie for nearly forty minutes and talked to Dave the entire time. I told him everything about my day.

When Sadie and I returned home, I turned on the TV for the first time since Dave and I watched *The Accountant* the night he said he felt like watching a movie, that Saturday night before he never left the bed again. I tried my best to give my brain a break and focus on whatever was playing. It didn't really work.

As I got ready for bed, I stood in the bathroom having my nightly conversation out loud with Dave, or myself, I'm not sure which. Mostly I told Dave how much I miss him and love him. The words "I miss you" are still scribbled in lipstick on Dave's side of the bathroom mirror.

As I came to a close in the relatively short conversation, I had a thought that in some way was the tiniest bit comforting: I will never in my lifetime be sadder than I am right now.

Tuesday, November 14

This morning I headed out to the allergist to get my weekly shot, followed by a visit to our safety deposit box. I need to probate the will so I needed the original. While in the little room at the bank, I rifled through the green folder I've kept up to date over the years for anyone who might have had to take care of wrapping up Dave's and my life should something have happened to us simultaneously. It has our medical proxies, wills, Dave's life insurance policy, and a list of every account number that pertains to us. I grabbed the whole folder knowing it will still be quite some time before I can throw out anything of Dave's . . . even his medical proxy, which I clearly don't need any longer.

Realizing I was completely overdue for an oil change, I stopped into our regular place to get it done along with the usual tire rotation. I had a feeling they were going to tell me the air filter was filthy. I usually tell them to leave it and I'll have my husband do it. I'm quite proficient at home repairs and working on our camper, but I hate car stuff. Today I told them to change the filter.

As I drove home planning what kind of a special dinner Claire and I could have on her last night here, I got a call from her. She asked me if I could take her to the airport tonight and then stuttered and stammered for at least fifteen seconds. She seemed to go on forever without actually saying anything. I could tell something very wrong had happened. Turns out, Margaret was being rushed to the hospital, and Claire needed to get on a flight tonight. I told her I'd be home in less than ten minutes.

After I got home and Claire booked her flight, I asked her to fill in the gaps. She told me that last night Margaret had been playing her usual game of tennis with the girls. While she was playing, she froze up several times on the court. Each time this happened, she had a flashback of the four of us—herself, Patrick, Dave, and me—during Dave's last days. She apologized to her lady friends for her bizarre actions; they certainly understood she was grieving the death of her brother.

Now I've said before that Margaret and Claire are the two smartest women I've ever known on the planet. Margaret has a résumé and academic credentials that if written on her arms would run all the way up one and down the other. Having never been a mother, she's an extremely doting aunt to seven very lucky nieces and nephews, always taking an extreme interest in their lives and the lives of their children. Basically, Margaret is a female version of Dave. Being a certified thanatologist, she's not afraid of anything death-related, never has been, and has sat with several people when they crossed over. She's always been my go-to person when one of my dogs has died.

Apparently, today Margaret was running a meeting at work and suddenly forgot who she was and what she was doing. The paramedics were called, as was Claire. When Claire got on the phone with Margaret, Margaret didn't know who Claire was. So as not to agitate Margaret, paramedics got her off the phone, and two people from work rode to the hospital with her. Being that Margaret is as beloved as Dave was at work, her associates are more like extended family than work folk.

As I drove Claire to the airport, she was getting texts that Margaret didn't know Dave had died. When she was told he had, she kept looping through the same series of questions: "Dave's dead? How did he die? Where is Patty? Where are the kids? How did I get here? Why am I here?" The doctors have confirmed she did not have a stroke and are running more tests.

If I were a gambling woman, I would bet Margaret was having a severe trauma response and her brain was protecting her from what she was suddenly unable to process. I called Margaret's sister, who happens to be a nurse, to inform her as well as Patrick. He's the only other person who knows what we went through.

After Claire was safely on the plane, I called out to Dave. I told him that although I would love to have him with me all day, every day, and to keep flooding me with signs, he now needs to go be with Margaret. He needs to help his sister through this. I will certainly be a mess for a while, so after Margaret is on the mend he can come back and help me work through my grief.

Thursday, November 16

Last night when I got ready for bed, I had my usual conversation with Dave. The bathroom is very triggering for me . . . something to talk to Mandy about. A lot of bad things happened in the bathroom, but we also had our Tub Talks there, so there's that.

I know I still have a lot of anger pent up, and I might have gotten out just a touch of it last night. As I stood in front of Dave's side of the vanity, thinking back to every moment that took place right in that spot, I found myself gripping the sink and rocking back and forth. I'm a little surprised I didn't loosen the entire thing from the wall. But the part that surprised me the most was that I let out the most guttural sound from my throat I have ever heard come out of my body. It was the kind of sound you can make only when alone in the house with the windows closed or someone would call the police. I felt completely numb afterward. Without a tear, I walked into the bedroom and climbed into bed.

Since I've loaned Dave out to Margaret for a couple of days, I asked him if he would visit me in a dream. People say you can do that. It all seems a bit hokey to me, but it's really all I have right now.

I woke up at 5 a.m. to use the bathroom. Realizing I didn't dream of Dave, I mumbled, "You didn't come to me in my dreams, Dave." I fell back to sleep and woke about an hour later, realizing I'd just dreamed of Dave. It wasn't awful, but it was heartbreaking.

I'm thinking about the Find My app on my phone. When I open the app, it shows Dave is at home because his phone now lives on the kitchen counter. Moments later, I'm sitting in a hospital with him. I can't see him, but I know he's sitting on a chair in the doctor's office. He has to go for scans and leaves the room ahead of me because I have to do something—I think I'm putting on my shoes. I know he's one hallway ahead of me, and I know he's with Megan. I can't catch up. I pull out my phone to open the Find My app and can't get the phone to work. I finally do, then realize the app is going to show him at home . . . because he is dead now.

That was my thought as I woke from the dream. Just a horrible way to start the day.

Some folks tell me the fact that I'm actually able to get out of bed, shower, eat some breakfast, tidy the house, and walk the dog is an amazing feat during this early state of grieving. I hear many people can't even get out of bed. I'm sure anyone looking in from the outside would think I'm getting along just fine. But instead of being on the constant highs and lows of the roller coaster, I'm now on a merry-go-round. I just go round and round. Same shit, different day. No emotional variety. No highs, no lows. As my friend Chris-from-the-beach says, "Rinse and repeat." It's like someone has taken all the color out of my world and it's now just black and white.

*   *   *

To start today's tasks, I first drove to the coffee shop. What a surprise . . . Jeremy and Tracey were there. I rarely catch them at the same time. Jeremy came around the counter to hug and kiss me like he does every time I see him, while Ashley grabbed my protein drink to make my special concoction. Jeremy shouted out, "Patty is now the only member of the Free Coffee for Life Club. David and I talked about that; his membership conveys to her."

Jeremy mentioned this to me the other day, so I asked him, "Did you and Dave really talk about that?" He insisted they had. A smirk formed on my face as I thought of Dave getting a laugh by making sure Jeremy wasn't going to get away scot-free without giving someone free coffee for life.

After grabbing some free coffee, I made the one-hour drive to speak with an attorney to make sure I'm probating the will correctly. He said I'm doing everything right. After I left, I tended to a few errands since I don't get down to Wilmington much lately. I put Trader Joe's in the GPS on my phone to find the easiest way to get there from the attorney's office. Never going there from this end of town, it took me an unfamiliar way: right through Old Town Wilmington, right past the house Dave and I stayed at when we came the weekend of Thanksgiving 2013 to scout out the place for our retirement. A flood of memories poured through me.

Thankfully, I got word that Margaret is being discharged from the hospital today. Much of her memory has returned. There's absolutely nothing physically wrong with her. The entire episode had been driven by grief and trauma. The power of the brain is incomprehensible.

31

Friday, November 17

*T*wenty-two years ago today was my thirty-seventh birthday. It was a Saturday.

Dave has planned a night in New York City, complete with dinner and a Broadway show. Quite possibly this night will give us more laughs in the future than we could imagine.

Dave takes me to a little French restaurant. It's cute, chic, and underground. The tables are close together, as they often are in most NYC restaurants. Our table has an upholstered bench seat that runs along the wall side and a chair on the other. It's presumed the lady will take the bench seat and her male companion will take the chair. It's an intimate setting but not private; the table to my left is less than a foot away.

We peruse the menu. I see foie gras and I flinch. Dave doesn't know yet what an avid animal lover I am. I'm nauseated at the way foie gras is harvested and never frequent restaurants that serve it. Dave doesn't know that... yet.

Suddenly he pulls a small jewelry box out of his pocket. He opens the box and says, "I want to marry you."

Silence.

I'm extremely literal and thinking, "You didn't ask me a question."

Pause for twenty seconds.

"Yes. I will marry you."

Poor guy . . . I have no idea how nervous he is. He slides the perfect ring onto my finger, the one I picked out, and we embrace. The couple next to us applauds. Everyone loves the moment that a marriage proposal brings—all the hope, promise, and love of two people joining together to witness each other's lives and tackle the rest of the world, and the commitment to becoming the second member of a two-person team.

We go to the show and see Phantom of the Opera. *It's brilliant! Ultimately, it's my favorite show of all time. The story . . . the sadness . . . the love . . . the pain.*

I stare at my left hand all night, centering the perfect diamond that's on the perfect ring on my left ring finger. Dave jokes that he could have taken me to a movie considering how little of the show I watched.

Today is my fifty-ninth birthday and the first one I've spent alone in a very long time. It's also the anniversary of our engagement, a double whammy of firsts. Everyone talks about the "firsts": the first Christmas without him, the first Thanksgiving without him . . . good Lord, the list goes on and on. There are so many firsts that aren't "traditionally" significant, I can't even mention them all. I also have not yet discovered them all.

In keeping with my daily promise to Dave to do the best I can, I made plans to meet Nora for lunch at the coffee shop. I've picked up coffee and walked through the shop since Dave died, but I still haven't sat at a table. And I have no intention of sitting at "our" table today.

I met Nora at 11:30. As we approached the counter, I didn't recognize the girl who was going to take our order. I knew everyone there except for some of the summer help, and I saw Ashley busy as always. Since we were ordering lunch, something I don't ordinarily do there, I needed to look at the menu. When the girl handed one to me, I noticed that inside her right forearm was a fairly large tattoo of a butterfly with one red wing and one blue wing. The year 1999 was written above it.

I didn't hesitate for a second in asking her, "Why do you have that tattoo?"

She said it's the year she was born.

"Why the blue and red butterfly? What's the significance?" I asked.

"None," she said. "I just like it."

Figuring she thought I was a bit demanding at this point, I told her my husband recently passed and I'd worn a dress with red and blue butterflies all over it. She wasn't particularly moved.

Nora and I ordered lunch and sat at a table. The second we sat down I heard the Christmas playlist coming out of the speakers. "Merry Christmas, Darling" started playing. This song has made me cry even on my happiest of days, and I couldn't believe it was playing. Then I listened to the lyrics about being apart but still "Christmasing" together. I started wondering whether I may have received two signs from Dave.

When the girl with the butterfly tattoo walked past our table, I stopped her to ask if I could take a picture of her tattoo and ask how long she's worked there. She told me since September. No wonder I don't know her; she started only a month before Dave died.

Nora and I ate lunch. I cried on her shoulder. She made me an adorable bandana for Sadie that says, "Tits my mom's birthday." Nora always gets in a laugh.

When we left the coffee shop, I planned to keep the forward momentum going by changing clothes and going to pet the horses. I'm extremely proud of myself for taking this step towards being proactive in my healing.

I texted my riding instructor to let her know I was coming by. She had plenty of time to talk and didn't have a lesson for hours. As I was driving, Celine Dion's "Because You Loved Me" came on the radio, the song Dave selected and we played while the family walked into the memorial service at the church.

It was great getting a little horse therapy, but I was sad to learn my riding instructor is moving on. She'll only take students interested in showing, and that's not a match for me. When Dave was still here, I told him I'd stopped my riding lessons but that I'd go back to the horses later . . . after . . . But now I don't know how that's going to happen. I guess if it's meant to be, it will work out somehow.

Three signs today? Did I get three signs today or a whole lot of coincidences? Why don't I let myself believe they're signs? There's no harm in doing that.

*   *   *

My family and friends were wonderful in reaching out today to send love and birthday wishes. Phone calls, texts, cards, gifts . . . everyone is doing their best to help me feel less alone.

My last call of the day was from Megan. I was surprised and quite pleased that she sounded like she was doing far better than I thought she would. Since she appeared strong, I let myself be weak and share how my heart is hurting. We talked about Christmas, and I told her that while I know her dad would want me to come to her house, I'm not sure if the logistics will work. She provided me more relief than she knows by telling me she'd spoken with her dad when she was last here, and he'd said that the first Christmas after . . . Patty would want to be alone, then by the following one she would return to family. Dave knew me so well.

When I told Megan I've been concerned with WWDD, she said, "Dad would want you to do what makes you feel best."

She was absolutely right! I've been so concerned about disappointing him, even though I know his first concern would be doing what's in my best interest. This may be just what I needed to hear to cut myself some slack.

Before the day ended, I thought about taking a tub. I haven't been in the tub since my Tub Talks with Dave. This is as difficult a step as sitting in the coffee shop, and for a few minutes I thought maybe I was doing too much in one day. I trusted my heart and filled the tub. It was a no-brainer deciding to sit on the side with the plumbing instead of the side with the smooth porcelain.

How can it be only weeks ago that I sat there burning his image into my brain while his head was leaning back against the blue, rubber pillow? I'd tried to memorize everything about those moments so I could bring them back to life when he was no longer here.

It was painful but also minimally comforting. I spoke out loud and pretended Dave was here. I told him about the horses, how I'm doing the best I can with my days, and how I remember twenty-two years ago today he told me he wanted to spend the rest of his life with me . . . and he did.

32

Sunday, November 19

I'm baffled by the way my days have changed from bouncing from project to project and place to place weeks before Dave's dying to spending seemingly never-ending days that sprawl out before me. Naturally when hospice became involved, my days became consumed with living the role of caregiver. However, it seems it was a very short time before then that I had a normal life of running to appointments, going to the grocery store and the gym, visiting and riding horses, and starting new projects on my camper.

The thing about grief is that it steals your will to do any of that. Now I have all the time in the world. From the moment I wake up to the moment I go to sleep, I'm accountable to no one except Sadie. People tell me I need to be patient with myself. I've never been patient with myself. If I were half as patient with myself as I was with Dave, well . . . that would be amazing.

Last night I completed a form online to donate a holiday wreath from Wreaths Across America. They will be placing wreaths on veterans' graves on December 16 in the cemetery where Dave is buried. There's an option of either placing the wreath on your beloved's grave personally or letting one of the volunteers do it. Naturally, I want to place the wreath on Dave's grave myself. I also agreed to volunteer several hours that day to help place as many wreaths as needed. It will be my honor. I reached out to Colonel Tom to see whether he might like to join me. No surprise, he does. Volunteering is not new to me, and I've always believed one of the ways to help yourself is by helping others.

After picking up my coffee today, I drove to the cemetery. I needed to see where Dave's body is buried. On the way, I tried to make a mental shift by not saying "where Dave is buried." Dave was a beautiful, intellectual, clever, generous, trustworthy, and loving soul. There is no way Dave is buried anywhere. There is no way his light could have just gone . . . out. There is no way Dave is "dead-dead" or "over-over." I wrestle with that idea daily due to my lifelong fears of death. But I know one thing for sure: The body I saw in that box on November 3 is *not* my Dave.

When the VA sent me the documents finalizing Dave's headstone, they also sent me maps of the cemetery. Since the service wasn't graveside, I had no idea where his body was. All I knew was G-106, which made me think of a Bingo board. Who would think your final resting place would conjure up images of a Bingo board?

I took Sadie for the ride and followed the map to section G. Before getting out of the car, I put the leash on her because her sprinting across the graves of others would be disrespectful. I started looking for the last row of G and then counted over eight graves. *One . . . two . . . three . . . four . . . five . . . six . . .* I could see in the distance where the sod was changing. At grave number six was mature sod, at number seven grass seed that recently sprouted, and at eight . . . straw and dirt.

My heart was pounding. I saw the back side of a temporary grave marker on number eight. Dave's grave is the start of a new row. There's already an occupied grave beside him with a temporary marker that resembles the stick that arrives in a flower bouquet so the sender can attach a name card. Although, this marker had a frame around the card, so it wouldn't blow away, I imagine. I walked to the front side of the marker and stood to the side of the grave.

David J. Gilbride

Oh my God! This is real! He's actually buried here.

I sat smack in the middle of the grave while staring at the marker and crying loudly. There was no need to worry about someone hearing me there. It's a place where people are allowed to let their pain flow, to let their unused love run out of their bodies in the form of tears. It should be obvious to any witnesses that I was beside the new graves and not the established ones . . . and that my grief is still raw.

Eventually, I walked Sadie to the edge of the cemetery where I could let her off-leash to run in the woods. We walked to the main road near the front entrance, then turned back the way we came. Before I got to where the graves begin, I re-leashed Sadie. We walked back to Dave's grave, and I lay on the narrow strip of grass right next to his grave. The sky was bright blue without one single cloud. My mind drifted, wondering whether Dave is a light somewhere in the universe or his light has been snuffed out forever. The whole idea was too overwhelming. I told him again how much I love him, that I will love him forever, then Sadie and I headed back to the car.

Later in the day, Jeremy and Tracey called me. They travel constantly, and it seems they're often going to and from the airport when they call. I know they're concerned about me. Actually, I'm quite fortunate to have many people who are concerned about me. Jeremy asked what I'm doing this Thursday. It's Thanksgiving. I've been planning to stay home, just me, myself, and I. Oh, and Sadie. They want me to come for dinner to share the craziness of their large, blended family. In my head, I heard Dave telling me to go. "There's always plenty of time for crying. Go have dinner with our friends," he would say. I told them I would join them, and Jeremy asked me to bring my éclair cake. Yes, Jeremy, I will bring an éclair cake.

Monday, November 20

Today was the first time I've spoken with Margaret since before she was rushed to the hospital. I was afraid I would unintentionally hurt her with my words. I didn't want to trigger her, as Claire told me Margaret was afraid she would cry when we talked. Geez. I told her that's the last thing she has to worry about. I cry all the time! I told her it's love leaking out . . . when you have so much love for someone you lost, that love has nowhere to go, so it squirts out your eyes.

When we spoke, I learned she's afraid she has let me down. Let me down? How could she be afraid she let me down? She was solid as a rock when she was here. From the moment she arrived days before Dave's death through the week following his funeral, she never wavered. No way did she let me down! "Of course, it would've been nice if you hadn't slept like a rock and I didn't have to wing a jar of ointment down the hall to wake you," I told her. We both shared a laugh.

I told Margaret about some of the signs I've been receiving. I'm still on the fence about believing in signs, but I did have a dream that was much better than the nightmare I had weeks ago.

> *Dave is whole again, with his round face and his round belly. He's shopping at a clothing store, pulling clothes on hangers off racks and flopping the articles across his arm. He goes into the dressing room and comes out wearing three shades of blue: blue pants, a blue T-shirt, and a blue button-down shirt. He stands waiting for my approval. I laugh and tell him he hasn't learned anything about the color wheel.*

Dave appearing whole in the dream suggests he is now pain-free. And it's funny as hell that he wore three shades of blue. Dave was always putting on a green shirt with blue pants and asking if the colors worked. After years of this, I finally told him to look at the color wheel. "Look at blue and go directly across from it. What do you see? Red, orange, yellow … perfect colors to complement blue." I think it's hilarious that in my dreams he still hasn't mastered the color wheel. But in truth, he was getting quite good at it!

Margaret told me that her sister, Ann, had an interesting dream too.

> *Ann and Margaret are standing on the edge of land next to a waterway of some sort. Dave is kayaking, looking young and handsome with his brown hair and muscles. Ann says it's how he looked in his thirties. He's paddling in some extremely rough water, then turns, and all they see is his back as Dave paddles away from them on water smooth as glass. He calls to them and says, "It was really rough going for a while there, but it's smooth sailing now."*

33

Saturday, November 25

This morning I returned to my favorite yoga class. I haven't been to the gym in about six weeks, and I need to get my body moving again. Walking Sadie is just not going to be enough.

The class was sparsely populated today. I suppose people are still traveling for Thanksgiving weekend. I was a regular at this class for many, many months and then stopped coming in early July, first because of the increased summer traffic, then because we were out of town for BLT 2023, then Dave got sick, then . . .

The instructor saw me, she said how good it was to see me again. I closed the physical gap between us and said, "My husband was very sick and he died four weeks ago tomorrow." As I spoke, my eyes welled with tears, as did hers. She asked if she could hug me and was visibly upset.

I always said that when I retired I was going to learn yoga. What I didn't know is that you don't "learn yoga," you "practice yoga." It's always practice, never perfection. That's a difficult concept for me. And most yoga classes, in my experience, begin with setting an intention. I've never liked setting an intention. Basically, I intended to get through this class by focusing only on my body and my form and not comparing myself to anyone else. Every class I set the same intention. But today the class started with lying back on the mat on blocks and stretching out the front of our bodies. The music was slow and sort of melancholy. My Achilles' heel in yoga has always been these slow, reflective moments. As my chest was pressed up to the sky, I heard the instructor say, "Open your heart."

That did it. Two streams of tears, one from each eye, started running down the sides of my face towards my temples. As my tears fell to the mat, I started thinking about when I first started yoga. It was an awful time in my life, certainly second to my current pain, but it was the worst I'd experienced up until that point in my life.

It was late summer of 2015. Dave and I had been married for thirteen years, and both of us had just retired. We were both going through some growing pains. Although exciting, leaving our jobs was a major change for both of us. We'd both been working since we were thirteen years old. Moving several states away was also difficult, probably more so for me since the house we were moving away from was the only house I'd ever owned. I'd bought it as a single woman when I was thirty, put lots of sweat equity into it, and owned it exactly twenty years to the day when we sold it. Dave and I were having some personal issues as well. I didn't really know what they were, but they kept popping up and we both kept pushing them down. It was hard for fix-it people like us to deal with something when we couldn't put our finger on the problem.

The last months of 2015 were very tumultuous for Dave and me. We decided shortly before Christmas we needed to separate for a while. It wasn't a separation with the intention of divorce but with the intention of figuring out what was going on and how to make it better, whether that be together or apart.

Dave moved to Florida on New Year's Eve. Megan was living down there with her family, so it seemed a sensible place for him to go. He was always a doting grandpa, just the way he was always a doting dad. Dave got settled in with a job to keep him busy and a place to live. I stayed here in our beautiful beach house with my dog at the time, named Piper. All those sayings about love being what makes a house a home are so true. A beautiful house is just a beautiful house when there's no love inside the walls.

I was still figuring out retirement and trying to keep busy with both a cycling group and a dance class I'd joined. When I wasn't doing those things, I was hanging out with Piper on the beach. I was also working on getting the hang of yoga, attending classes at the local community center a couple of times a week. At the end of the class, we'd lie in a position called "Savasana," or the final resting pose. This is a time to lay flat on the mat with your eyes closed and your arms gently lying next to your body, palms facing the sky. Your mind should be empty. No one talks about it, but "Savasana" actually translates to "death pose" or "corpse pose." It's a time to let your body and mind reap the benefits of your practice and just let go of whatever no longer serves you. Then you roll to one side in the fetal position and are reborn.

I was not comfortable with any of this. Death pose? Nope. Petrified of dying. Let your mind go? Nope. My mind never shuts off.

The only way I could come close to letting my mind go was to create a little visualization. I'd imagine I was walking to the beach with Piper. No one else was on the beach. I'd lay a fringed blanket on the sand and lie on it, telling Piper to lay down and wait for me. The blanket would rise straight up like a magic carpet, with Piper lying directly under it. The sky was blue, the sun was warm on my face, and the gulls were singing their songs. While I was still lying on the blanket, it would glide directly over the ocean where it would then hover. Eventually the blanket glided back over Piper and onto the beach. As it lowered, Piper would get up and wait for me to lower and settle. I would praise her and fold up the blanket, and we'd leave the beach together. This is the only way I could get through Savasana without thinking about my separation from Dave, my retirement, my changing life. Thank God Savasana is no longer than two minutes.

On February 21, just shy of two months after Dave left, I was doing a jigsaw puzzle on the dining room table, trying to keep my mind off other things. Piper was lying on the front porch.

I hear a neighbor walking up the steps, so I look out the front door. Piper is no longer on the porch. My neighbor stammers something about Piper . . . a car . . . down the street. I run past her and race to where I see a group of people gathered and a car parked off to the side. Everyone is standing around Piper. She's lying on the sidewalk as I run to her. She is dead.

Since Dave moved to Florida, Piper has been the only thing I have to love. She's been the only reason to get up in the morning, and now she is gone.

My neighbor's husband carries her back to my house and for hours digs a hole in the hard ground. I lie on the concrete under my house with Piper in my arms the entire time. I love hard and have trouble letting go.

After we bury her, I go into the house and call Dave. I don't remember the conversation at all. I also text Pastor Bobby, who I've known only for a few months. I tell him I'm not coming to church anymore. Within minutes, Bobby shows up at my door. I tell him, "God is not allowed in this house any longer. He's ruined my life. He doesn't care about me and I'm done with Him. God can stay in His house and I will stay in mine."

At night when I go to bed, I cry that I don't want to wake up in the morning. Weeks pass, and I eventually return to

yoga class. I get through the quiet moment at the begin-
ning by setting an intention, follow the class learning new
poses, then it's time for Savasana. My visualization with
Piper and the magic carpet has been my survival skill. It's
the only way I know how to get through Savasana. The
tears stream down my face, so many they run into my ears
and make my hair wet. I dry my face before Savasana is
over and the rest of the class opens their eyes.

As the tears streamed down my face at the start of today's class, I wondered whether I'd be able to get through the rest of it. I kept thinking how the visualization of Piper and the magic carpet was just a distraction from the biggest issue at that time in my life: I was without my husband . . . my team-mate on a two-person team . . . my person.

The class was great, but I can feel I haven't been there in months and my muscles have weakened. The steady flow of poses kept my brain focused on the class . . . until Savasana. I didn't know how to get through that pose without crying. I thought about something completely different just to make the minutes pass.

As I walked to my car after class, I recalled this was always a time I would send a text to Dave saying, "Coffee?" He would answer with an enthusiastic, "Sure!" and then meet me at the coffee shop with Sadie. It was our norm every Saturday. I have crying jags constantly now, but this is going to be a big one . . . every Saturday after yoga.

I stopped by the coffee shop on the way home to get my drink to go. The girls' warmth and affection always make me feel welcome. I heard someone shout out, "Get shots ready! Patty is here." I don't have quite the rock-star status Dave had, but the recognition was heartwarming. I stayed for a few moments after getting my drink, then headed home for an appointment.

Bobby and I met for a walk after that. He and I have walked the beach before, talking about the town, local politics, family, his church, and of course, God. Bobby was ten minutes early today. The wind kicked up, so I threw on another jacket and suggested we walk the neighborhood streets because the beach was too cold and windy.

For two hours we walked and talked. We probably covered well over six miles, the first two of which I talked before Bobby even got a word in. He didn't jump right to talking about God, which is one of the things I like about him. He has always said he has more faith in my walk with God than I do. He loves that I continue to ask questions of God.

Why did I sail through the first fifty years of my life with barely a scratch, yet in the last eight years I separated from my husband, my dog was suddenly killed, and my husband got cancer and died? Each of those things is really big! What's going on? Why is this all happening now? Doesn't God like me?

I talked about Dave a lot. We talked about Dave's thoughts on God, faith, and dying, about his personality, and about what he added to this world and what he added to my life. I love talking about Dave! It warms my heart. I know no one will ever forget him, but somehow talking about him makes me feel like he's not so dead.

I told Bobby I often say "WWDD" when dealing with emotional issues. Dave was so good at dealing with my emotions. And unlike me, who was often impatient, hasty, and cared more about how I felt in the moment rather than considering the long run, Dave considered all angles.

As Bobby and I continued to talk, I ran through some of the more difficult relationships in my life. We spoke about how Dave taught me that while there are things I wish I could say to those people that would make me feel better in the moment, to what end would that lead? Ultimately, it would only make the other person feel bad, then I'd feel bad, and what would I have accomplished? I wouldn't resolve a problem, and I might actually create a new one. And what about when the day comes that I have my "life review," the passing through my mind of every action I've ever taken before I die? You hear a lot about life reviews when you start reading books about NDEs and when hospice comes into your life. When the day comes that I have my life review and look back at these moments, if I've hurt people I care about unnecessarily, I will regret having not handled it better. I'm sure Dave would agree that the right answer is not to confront them.

When I came home from our very long walk, I searched Google for quotes regarding personal growth occurring only during times of difficulty. I came across this quote from C. S. Lewis, and it resonated with the questions I asked Bobby:

> Imagine yourself as a living house. God comes in to rebuild that house. At first, perhaps, you can under-stand what He is doing. He is getting the drains right and stopping the leaks in the roof and so on; you knew that those jobs needed doing and so you are not surprised. But presently He starts knocking the house about in a way that hurts abominably and does not seem to make sense. What on earth is He up to? The explanation is that He is building quite a different house from the one you thought of—throwing out a new wing here, put-ting on an extra floor there, running up towers, mak-ing courtyards. You thought you were being made into a decent little cottage: but He is building a palace. He intends to come and live in it Himself.[3]

I continue to cry at least a dozen times each day over the loss of Dave. I miss him desperately! A tiny bit of me wonders if I can somehow grow from this experience, and if somehow that would make Dave smile.

Wednesday, November 29

I saw Mandy on Monday. I've always found a good therapist is an incredibly useful tool. Being that she's known me for eight years, she has an inside read on my playbook. She thinks my brain is spinning and spinning looking for something to fix. Courtesy of OCD, I have some perfect traits for being an advocate for a cancer patient, as I'm someone who never stops thinking about solving not only current problems but problems that don't yet exist but may in the future.

That's definitely what my brain did when Dave was still here. My brain just spun and spun with all the little issues that came up on a weekly basis until I could come up with a way to make a problem less of a problem. Sometimes Dave would even say, "Would you stop solving my problems?" Chuckle.

I've spent the last few days trying to give my overactive brain other chores: Get the truck inspected, get a haircut, take care of finances . . . it's just not enough. I need a problem to fix.

Walking Sadie on the beach tonight, I looked out at the vastness of the ocean. Not a soul was in sight. I asked Dave out loud, "How much time do I have left? One year or twenty?" Then I wondered how I would live my life differently based on the answer.

34

Saturday, December 2

*H*onestly, life is still pretty miserable. I just don't know how to respond to people when they ask how I'm doing. Mandy has suggested not thinking about the future, which is too overwhelming right now, and the idea of this feeling of grief lasting for a year or two is . . . well . . . unbearable.

I read a statistic the other day that the average age a wife becomes a widow is fifty-nine. I've always visualized widows to be little old ladies. I asked my newly widowed friend Chris-from-the-beach what she thinks of this statistic, being that she was fifty-seven when widowed. She said other than three who lost their young husbands to sudden deaths, all her friends were still coupled up. Then she asked about my friends.

For starters, I was fifty-eight when Dave died. My friend Joan, who's been walking my dog, was forty-nine. Diane was forty and Sheila was forty-eight. Maybe . . . yeah, maybe those ages are enough to drop the average age dramatically. And I thought being a widow at my age was going to be an anomaly. Turns out I'm just average.

I've started reading a little before bed, just long enough until my sleeping pill starts to take effect. Dave loved to read, but unfortunately reading became difficult for him with some of the physiological issues he was having. It was rather ironic that he couldn't read when he had all the time in the world. It reminded me of the *Twilight Zone* episode "The Obsolete Man" with Burgess Meredith. Cruel irony.

Having never been an avid reader, I'm particular about what I read. I have difficulty keeping my attention in the book; it's that damn spinning brain of mine that's the problem. Dave certainly didn't have that issue. I used to say to him, "Get out of the book, I'm talking to you." The house could have shaken and he'd be unaware if he were reading a book. But I've finished two books, and I remembered I have the perfect book to read next.

It's spring of 2022, and Megan has a great idea. She subscribes to a service called Storyworth that sends subscribers a question every week for a year about their lives, experiences, thoughts, and opinions. They can respond to the standard, prewritten questions, or they can write their own. Dave does both.

Every week when Dave receives a new question, he ponders it for a few days and then writes a few paragraphs. He submits all his responses back to the Storyworth website to be assembled for a future book. He has always enjoyed writing, and since Megan and I get to write questions and see his responses immediately, his stories make for great conversation the whole year. It's such a great way to discover things about each other that we never would have known otherwise. And it's certainly a terrific keepsake! Even I learn things about Dave, such as the reason he loves Payday bars. It's not just because they taste great but because they connect him to a memory he has of his dad in his youth.

At the time Dave starts this one-year project, he doesn't believe he will actually be able to finish it. He thinks the book will be printed and distributed posthumously.

Thankfully, Dave is able to proudly see the completion of the book and its distribution to key people. After the books are printed, I tell Dave, "You need to autograph my book." He smiles and whips out some silly remark. I never give it a second thought.

Dave's book, *There and Back Again*, has been lying on the coffee table for several months now. Tonight I grabbed my copy and brought it to bed with me to read again. As I opened the cover, I saw that I never reminded him to autograph it.

Saturday, December 2

I'm going to try to alter my routine today so I don't have that heavy reminder after Saturday morning yoga that my usual "Meet Dave and Sadie for coffee" is not happening anymore. That's how I handled change when I quit smoking over twenty years ago—I changed all the habits and routines associated with it.

Yoga is good for my mind and my body, but as usual, I ran into difficulty with Savasana and some of the mood-evoking music. Today I listened to the slow, groaning lyrics of a song called "Bloodstream" by Stateless. They describe being so close to someone that it feels like you've inhaled them; you feel them behind your eyes and in your bloodstream. The lights were low for today's class, so it was easy to wipe away my tears without an audience.

After I left the gym, I stopped for coffee on my way to the nail salon for a pedicure. I didn't go to my favorite coffee shop but to somewhere on the way where I actually paid for my coffee. While I waited for my two shots of espresso to mix with my protein drink, I remembered the time I came to this shop in 2019.

The cycling club Dave and I join is mostly retirees, but I'm thoroughly impressed with how fit these folks are! The club has several rides on the calendar each week for all levels of fitness. When Dave rides with me, we join a group ride at a slightly slower pace than when I ride without him. One thing this group is consistent about, regardless of the pace of the ride, is that there's always a coffee stop midway! These folks ride hard, stop for coffee and socializing, then hit the bikes hard again for the ride home.

One day while taking a thirty-five- to forty-mile ride, we stopped at this particular coffee shop. Two of my favorite riders are Paul and Mitch. They both are at least fifteen years my senior, are far stronger riders than I am, and enjoy my "never give up" attitude. Paul lives near me, and we often drive the forty-five minutes in his truck to the start of the ride. Mitch always wears matching "kits," crazy cycling outfits that match from head to toe; we affectionately tease him about some of the crazy clothes he wears.

I stop riding with the group when my lower back issues become severe, but I stay in touch with Paul via text.

While sitting in the airport waiting to fly to Colorado, I hear my phone ring a few minutes before boarding. It's Paul. He says he has bad news. Mitch is dead. He'd been diagnosed with brain cancer about three months ago, and he just died. I'm speechless. I last saw him when we stopped at this coffee shop with the group. I'm stunned how something like that could happen so fast. I have no idea how my world will change fourteen months later with Dave's diagnosis.

After coffee, I stopped at the nail salon without an appointment and asked Nancy if someone had time to give me a pedicure. "Sure, seat number 3," she said. As I sat in the massage chair playing with the buttons, I looked at the young lady giving a pedicure to a woman in seat number 2. The pedicurist was wearing a blue T-shirt with butterflies on it, along with the words, "Be the Change." More blue butterflies . . .

Sunday, December 3

Today was my first lesson on horseback since July. Although my instructor is leaving, she said she'll be available for another month.

When I was a kid, I went to two weeks of "camp with horses," but we didn't have the money for me to take regular riding lessons. I've never thought of doing it as an adult, but in my fantasy life I'm a barrel-racing, cow-chasing cowgirl.

> *It's two summers ago, and Dave and I are driving to one of our last stops on the first BLT. We're in the truck, pulling the camper behind us. A bit earlier I'd done a little horseback riding at a friend's place in Montana. Driving and thinking for hours, I say to Dave, "I want a horse."*

> *Dave knows I would never make any decision impulsively, especially one that involves a living creature. However, for the next ten hours, while Dave is captive as my passenger, he gets to listen to me talk about horses.*

> *The following week, when we're settled in at home, I continue researching. I'm looking for a working ranch where I can work for a week to see if I can get this "I should have been born a cowgirl" and "I want a horse" thing out of my head. I don't want to vacation at a dude ranch; I want to spend time at a working ranch. With flights becoming so expensive over the last year, and with so many connecting flights having been dropped since the pandemic, I*

consider a ranch in Nebraska instead of Montana or Wyoming, which would have been my preference.

I can't plan anything too far in the future since Dave's health can change at any moment, but he seems to be in a healthy enough state right now that he'll be able to make his nutrition shakes himself with a little coaching from me ahead of time.

I make reservations for the first week of September. Oh my goodness, September 7 is our twentieth wedding anniversary, and I won't be here with Dave. This is a milestone anniversary! Starting to stress over this, I ask Dave his thoughts.

"We'll celebrate when you get home," he says. "It's just a date."

Off I go, flying into Omaha on a Sunday and renting a car to drive to Burwell, Nebraska, where I live the cowgirl life for a week.

The trip is great! We have a small group of about eight people and get to know each other quite well. We share all our meals and our days together with our hosts. Never having formal horseback riding lessons, I do okay and manage to sit on the horse I'm assigned for four to six hours a day. Every muscle in my body hurts, which Dave gets to hear about every evening when I talk to him on the phone.

On September 7, after my group returns to the barn and gets the horses untacked and fed, my host tells me there's a delivery in the main house for me. I head for the kitchen, where my host's wife points to my place setting at the long dining room table. I'm at least twenty feet away, but I can see there's a stuffed sloth propped on my plate. Dave's *spirit animal. My eyes well with tears as I immediately recognize the sloth is from my husband.*

I nuzzle the soft sloth and cry. I rush back to my cabin to call Dave. Naturally, being that I'd be in the middle of nowhere for our twentieth wedding anniversary, he started figuring out weeks ago what he was going to send and from where he was going to send it. Dave has always been thoughtful in this way.

When I return home, Sloth takes up a position on our bed with the decorative pillows and Gingerbread Man. Now we each have our spirit critter. Dave is represented by the extremely . . . slow . . . moving . . . sloth. And I am represented by, "Run, run, run as fast as you can, you can't catch me, I'm the gingerbread man."

Monday, December 4

This morning I woke up right after a dream about Dave.

We're in a restaurant. Our seafood platters arrive. Mine is a normal-sized portion; Dave's is huge—he has nearly every kind of seafood on the plate. He pushes the plate to the middle of the table, and I ask him what's wrong. He gives me that knowing look. I sadly say, "Oh, you're not hungry," realizing he only ordered food so that I would enjoy my dinner.

Suddenly he starts to choke and gag. His eyes bulge. I run around to his side of the table shouting, "Call 911!"

I realize as I get to him that I don't know what to do. I panic. He has a DNR . . . I can't let them start an airway. I feel like the sounds he's making aren't from choking on food but because this is the moment his body has decided to die. The couple of minutes waiting for EMS is a very long time to listen to Dave gagging and sputtering. How do I watch him suffer? How do I make him more comfortable? How do I stop this awful choking?

I think about all the people in the restaurant who will witness my husband die. Welcome to my world.

35

Tuesday, December 5

*W*hen Dave and I retired, we were bored to tears. I think Dave knew he wouldn't settle into retirement easily. Ultimately he took three jobs in the following years, so I suppose it was a good prediction. But when folks asked me what I was going to do, I said, "All the stuff I've wanted to do, but didn't have the time for."

Of course, moving to a new house in a new state and needing to make new friends was a huge undertaking at our ages. I've always thrived on a busy schedule; the busier, the better! After retirement, I'd knock out my to-do list first thing in the morning, then look at the clock at 10:17 a.m. and think, *What am I going to do with the rest of the day?*

It was my brother-in-law Tom, who retired years ahead of us, that gave us both some valuable advice. He said, "Instead of scheduling everything in one day, back-to-back, you need to spread things out over the course of a week. No more than one task per day." I think he was half joking, but it really was solid advice. I used Tom's method of easing into retirement until I got myself into a groove with a social circle, places to go, and things to do. I often find myself looking back at that advice and trying to put it into practice.

Prior to Dave's diagnosis, we'd been living in our new home for five years. Dave had started the town manager job, the third and final one after retirement, which he absolutely loved. I had my days all to myself and was really living my best life! I'd go to the gym, pick up a coffee, work in the garden, and walk the dog. Believing in the importance of volunteering, I trained one of our dogs to be a therapy dog. I'd drive an hour to volunteer with the hospital, hospice, or the advanced Alzheimer's facility. When I wasn't doing that, I was rescuing birds for the local bird sanctuary. I always loved to cook and bake, so a nice dinner was nearly always waiting for Dave, along with a tasty dessert. In all honesty, life couldn't have been better!

After cancer came into our lives, my schedule got a little crazier. It was never "undoable" in my mind, but I just kept adding things and rarely subtracting. Eventually there were doctors at the university hospital, doctors at the local hospital, infusions, research, prescriptions, and the constant enhancement of Dave's nutrition shakes, which I exhaustively researched. Still, I could be out running errands with a to-do list a mile long, but if at any time I looked at my phone and saw a text from Dave saying, "Coffee?" I would change my entire morning to spend quality time with him. That little one-word text was my husband asking me out on a date. I always replied with a resounding yes, knowing there would come a day when there would be no more coffee dates.

The job of a caregiver is a very gradual process. You don't realize how much of your mental, emotional, and physical self you're dedicating to it, nor how much of you you're losing. You feel like you're adding things because you're so busy, but really you're losing yourself. The emotional toll, especially on a person who tends to always seek control like me, is relentless. The constant push and pull of feeling like you're actually beating cancer and then falling into defeat is like a gut punch every time; like a failure. And every time it happens, it takes about one day—just one day—of feeling weak and scared before I pull on my Wonder Woman cape and target whatever issue has come our way. The roller coaster then shifts from the downward roar of defeat to a gentle climb of hope again.

That's how I survived for three years. Now it's all over. The fight is over. And I find that the twenty-four hours that exist in the course of a day are far longer than I ever remember them being.

So, I think back to Tom's words. Instead of tiptoeing out of bed while Dave sleeps, I sleep until 7 a.m. Instead of grabbing my computer and coffee and sitting on the couch so as not to disturb Dave, I crawl back into bed with coffee in hand, and Sadie joins me. Around 9 a.m., I finally get up to make my second cup of java or some breakfast. By the time I tidy up the house and walk Sadie on her much-longer-than-usual walk, it's 11 a.m. I've almost made it till noon. I look at the day in blocks of time. Hopefully, I have a chore or an appointment scheduled later in the day. If not, I write in my journal for an hour or two. Dave used to nap at 2:30 in the afternoon for a couple of hours, so I'd use that quiet time for journaling. At 4:30 or 5, Dave would wake and we'd start our evening routine together.

This has become an incredibly difficult time of day. How do I bridge the gap between 5 p.m. and when David Muir comes on the world news at 6:30 p.m.?

I've never been a big drinker. Back when Dave was healthy, we used to have an adult beverage on Friday. I called it "Cocktail Friday" for years and would have fun cooking new tapas recipes for us. I intentionally avoided alcohol immediately following Dave's death. With my dad dying of alcoholism when he was only forty-five years old, I'm very aware of substance abuse. Then, of course, there are my control issues, so I don't like the feeling of being drunk. But tonight I thought, *What the hell? I'll start having a daily shot of my favorite rock and bourbon every day at 5 p.m., if only to make my brain a little fuzzy to get me to the evening news. To dull the fact that Dave is not here.*

I didn't even put the news on for several weeks following Dave's death. I found it too upsetting. It was something we did together. This is one of the "little firsts" no one talks about—the day-to-day things you used to do with your person that now you will do alone. I've started watching the news again. I anticipate all the key moments when Dave would have his personal commentary. We generally agreed on most things political, but we certainly had our differences. Even if I don't watch the news, I like the sound now; it's familiar . . . like when Dave was still here.

If I'm lucky, I can time my day so that dinner and dishes are done by 7 p.m. Then I stream two shows on television, just like when Dave was here. That gets me close to 9 p.m., when I do my nighttime routine, have my conversation with Dave, go through my meltdown—if I haven't done so already—and climb into bed around 9:30 with a sleeping pill and a book. By 10 p.m., the lights are out. If I'm lucky, I sleep through most of the night . . . usually not.

I tend to wake up for the day when the sun comes up. If I open my eyes and see it's light, I look at the clock. If it's dark, I push myself to go back to sleep. It's usually near 7 a.m. when I wake up for good. And then I do it all over again. Rinse and repeat. Every day, the same damned thing.

When I saw Mandy yesterday, she commented at the end of our session that she could see I'm making progress. I agree, except in all honesty, though I spend less time wondering whether ending my life is a viable option, as I said to her, "It's the difference between dragging 500 pounds around your neck versus 499 pounds."

Yes, 499 is better. But it's still immense and seems unendurable.

36

Wednesday, December 6

Sometime during early October, after Dave and I had watched our evening shows while sitting on the couch together, I gently climbed over him and turned around so we could have our nightly embrace and face-to-face talk. I wanted to get his opinion about something, though I was pretty sure I knew what Dave's reaction would be.

> *"I want your opinion on something. I'm thinking I may want to get a tattoo of a blue butterfly. Where on my body do you think I should get it?" I ask.*
>
> *"Well," he says, "first, you know I don't like tattoos, so I don't think you should get it at all. But since that's not what you're asking me, how 'bout the back of the shoulder? Or do you want to be able to see it?"*
>
> *"This is only going to be a small, little butterfly," I reply. "I'm thinking I should get it right over my heart because it's about you and love and that there's something after this."*
>
> *Dave seems pleased it's not going to be a tattoo the size of my hand and comments that a small butterfly will be nice. He knows his opinion is important to me, but we've agreed to disagree regarding tattoos. I've had one for*

about a year and a half. It's a fairly small image of a heart with a paw print on my left ankle.

I get a tattoo only if it's something I feel passionate about, but recently I've been relaxing my often-unattainable views on the body and perfection. I've spent so many years focusing on coloring my gray hair, making sure my nails were done, and forever obsessing over my body dysmorphia. Although I don't want to go through life looking like a total slob, I'm starting to realize the body is just a vessel for the good stuff. I've often said all my scars are like little battle wounds that I'm proud of. It shows that I haven't spent my life sitting on the sidelines watching others play but have been out on the field playing my hardest. Either that or it shows I'm a complete klutz.

Watching Dave's body change over the last few years has certainly had an impact on me, specifically during the last two weeks. I realize how insignificant our body appearance is compared to how we are as a person. It has nothing to do with how smart, kind, sensitive, caring, strong, thoughtful, or inspirational we are. Our bodies facilitate physical action. That's it. They enable the person who's on the inside to actually "be and do" for the world on the outside.

Naturally, I went online and purchased two different temporary tattoos of blue butterflies—because I overthink everything. I didn't put the first one on until the week after Dave died and a couple of days before the funeral. It was probably only a half-inch wide, and it wasn't visible with my dress. I placed it exactly where I'd told Dave I would: above my heart.

Weeks later I tried the other one. I loved the fact it had a shadow that made it appear as though it was in motion. I placed it inside my left forearm. I'm still not sold on the placement.

I think I need a really convincing sign from Dave to go through with this, like a billboard with a blue butterfly that says, "This is your sign, Patty." Okay, maybe not that obvious, but I have asked for a very specific sign from Dave. I've been asking for weeks. It was that book *Signs* that said I should be specific. If I get *that* sign, the tattoo will be definite.

*   *   *

Today has been a quiet day for the most part. I saw my trainer at the gym this afternoon. As soon as we started, she asked, "What are we focusing on today?" I told her, "Absolutely anything. Just keep me working my body and don't give me time to think."

As I headed home, something started me on a crying jag. It was a really wild ride, as usual; one minute I'm driving the car and thinking about jumping into the shower, and the next I'm sobbing uncontrollably because of some song, some thought, some memory . . .

I still tend to ask Dave for a sign whenever I get really emotional. I can't believe how many times I've now said to him, "Please send me something to let me know you're okay!" I must sound crazy. It's probably due to the O in OCD. Tonight I reminded him about the very specific sign I've been asking from him for weeks: a shell with a painted blue butterfly and some inspirational saying painted on the other side. Occasionally you see them around here, being that I live at the beach. They're similar to the more popular painted rocks. I found one back in February. It was painted with beautiful pastel colors on one side, and on the inside were the words BE FEARLESS. As a matter of fact, Claire found one while she was here, so it's not unheard of.

After I got home, I was sipping my rock and bourbon while sitting in the pink chair in the living room, trying to bridge the time like I do every afternoon. A text pinged from Nora; no words, just a picture of a mass of painted oyster shells. The shell right on top of the pile had a huge, blue butterfly painted on it.

"Omg! Where was that picture taken?!" I wrote back.

She was at the nail salon where her daughter gets her nails done. She offered to snag the shell for me, but just the fact she saw it and was able to send me a picture was enough. Because I'm so rigid with my black-and-white thinking, I wrestled with wondering whether this qualified as my undoubtedly sure-fire sign from Dave. Though it didn't have a saying on it, I would have been happy with almost any saying, such as "Believe," "I love you," "Have faith," or "You're loved"; it could have said a zillion different things.

I could just hear Dave saying, "Would you give me a break? I gave you another blue butterfly, and it's on a shell like you asked." I never told anyone I was looking for a shell with a blue butterfly as a sign, so this really could be amazing.

So tonight, when I had my nightly meltdown, it was a touch different. I was kinder to myself. I looked at myself in the mirror and spoke the way I'd console a friend: "You poor girl, this is so unfair." Actually, I sounded much like Shirelle, a.k.a. Mary Poppins. Maybe it's because of a poem that Molly sent me earlier today. The gist of the poem is that when you miss someone the most, remember how they loved you and do that for yourself; love yourself harder on those days. Maybe that's why today I've been just a bit gentler with myself.

And tonight, while I'm sitting here on the edge of the bed where I feel so close to Dave because we spent so much time here, I'm remembering how I always put my arm around him and pulled him close while I rested my head on his shoulder. I'm reminded of the scene in the movie *Ghost* when Demi Moore's character is at the pottery wheel and the ghost (played by Patrick Swayze) is sitting behind her with his arms around her, the song "Unchained Melody" by the Righteous Brothers playing in the background. I imagine, just for a moment, that Dave is here and I have my arm around him. I say a few things to him out loud and reply to myself with what I know his words would be. It brings me just a little peace tonight.

37

Thursday, December 7

I actually had three things on the calendar for this morning. In an effort to get back to taking care of my health, I had an appointment for fasting blood work first thing in the morning, followed by shopping with Cathy, then a massage at noon.

Cathy texted me last night. We're what I would call "casual friends." She told me she recently had eye surgery and asked if I could take her to the store to get a few things. She has a very strong Christian faith and said one thing in her text that seemed so odd to me. She said she was praying to the Lord about who to ask for help and the Lord brought me to her mind. I thought, *What a strange thing to ask God about.* But this is a win–win for both of us; I need to fill my days with worthwhile activities. Cathy also happens to be another friend who has experienced the death of her husband, in her case when she was only forty-seven years old, so I thought maybe she could give me insight into how she survived. Plus, if the Lord really did have something to do with putting my name in her head, the visit might be beneficial for both of us.

I arrived at my doctor's office with my coffee in hand and ready to drink as soon as I left. When I got called back to the phlebotomist's office, my doctor saw me walk by and stuck her head into the room. She knew Dave died and had called me several weeks ago to check on me. She gently rubbed my back and asked me how I was doing. That's all it takes these days. A lump formed in my throat and I couldn't speak. All I could do was shake my head and shrug my shoulders.

Unfortunately, since my patient folder isn't emblazoned with a scarlet "RW" for "Recent Widow," the other two ladies in the office didn't know of my recent loss. I've been trying to be more Dave-like and not blab to everyone that I just lost my husband.

Gal Number One asked me for my date of birth. Upon my telling her, she said, "Oh, you just had a birthday. Did you do anything fun?"

"Not really," I said in a low voice.

Then Gal Number Two said, "Are you all ready for the holidays?"

As I watched the vials fill with my blood, I started thinking how on par these questions were with the fact it felt like someone was draining the life out of me.

"As ready as I'll ever be," I replied.

Since I had to fast for this test, I was anxious to leave and run next door for a breakfast sandwich. As I ate, I got a phone call from the dentist's office. The voice on the other end of the phone said, "Hi, Mrs. Gilbride? We've been trying to call Mr. Dave's phone, but we keep getting a weird message that the calls aren't going through."

"That's because my husband passed away on October twenty-ninth. I canceled this appointment weeks ago," I replied.

I thought back to the day I scrolled through the calendar on my phone: Green is for me, yellow for Dave, red for any dog-related events, and purple for unshared events on my calendar. Yes, I know, very OCD. I went through all the yellow calendar events and changed or canceled them. I also unshared my calendar with Dave. I couldn't stand the fact that every time I added something to my calendar, Dave's phone would ding with the notification "Patty added a calendar event." This is the stupid, upsetting, frustrating stuff that happens. But it's the stuff that happens every day that draws attention to the fact that your person is no longer here. It all just kind of hit me, and I struggled to hold back the tears since I was still sitting in Dunkin'.

I texted Cathy and asked her if we could hang out for a bit before we went shopping since I had a tough morning. Turns out we talked for nearly two hours! Although we're of similar description, I never would have thought we have as many similarities in our lives as we do. Cathy isn't pushy with her faith, but it's what she believes in from the bottom of her soul, so she's passionate about it. I'm at a point where I'm questioning everything, and my usual black-and-white thinking still wants black-and-white answers. Although she couldn't provide that, we did have a thought-provoking conversation.

Cathy said she doesn't remember details of some of the awful things in her past and thanks God for His grace in helping her forget them. I find this such a strange way of thinking. I asked her, "Don't you think your brain is wired to forget painful memories, the same way a woman forgets the pain of childbirth before she's ready to have another child?" I was thinking about how my bathroom used to be such a relaxing room, but now I struggle every time I walk in because it's filled with so many painful memories. She suggested I get down on my knees and pray to God, asking Him to help lessen the load of the painful memories and let them be overcome with the remembrance of the sweet memories like the Tub Talks. I suppose it couldn't hurt.

All these questions, and neither one of us had or has the "right" answers. These are not black-and-white questions but questions that revolve around faith versus science. I've always relied on science because it's concrete. My OCD also commands certainty. I don't do well with any kind of faith, not just faith in God but faith in people. I learned at an early age that if you rely on only yourself, you will never be disappointed. That all changed with Dave. I had complete faith and trust in him. Quite honestly, he was the only person in the world I could say that about. With him gone, I'm back to relying totally on myself, but my mind is probably more open to other people's ideas now than it ever has been before.

This evening when I was all alone, I got down on my knees.

It's scary to be all alone in the world. My heart carries such a heavy load, and I don't know how I'm going to survive this. I don't really know how to pray, at least not like I've heard Cathy pray, and certainly not like Pastor Bobby prays. But tonight I asked God to take away all the bad memories in the bathroom. I went through each memory one by one, crying a little harder each time I brought up the next. I told Him of the night Dave said, "I don't want you to remember me like this." I asked for help to forget.

And then, before I was done, I said to Dave, "Just because God may be in the picture doesn't mean you're off the hook for sending me blue butterflies. Please send me more!" Amen.

38

Monday, December 11

*I*t's been a rough couple of days, mostly because I've been sick. I was doing great on Saturday; not like when I was living my best life, but under the circumstances it was a fairly decent day.

Sadie and I went on a nice long walk, then I spent a few hours working in the yard in the spring-like weather. I haven't given a hoot about my garden in months, so it's a good sign that I even cared to *think* about it. Not to mention, when I told Mandy I wanted to find a way to relieve my anger by destroying the crap out of something, she suggested using that energy in a positive way rather than a destructive one, such as working in the garden.

Although I have a high regard for Mandy's advice, I've done some reading and found a couple of "rage rooms" near me. It's on my list of things to do. Granted, I also read that letting loose with anger like that is known to increase anger rather than decrease it. But ever since Dave and I got on the cancer train, I've really wanted to beat the shit out of something. Now I've gotten sidetracked talking about anger . . .

After working in the yard, I took a nice hot shower and got into my comfy clothes. I noticed my throat was starting to feel sore. *Please God, no!* There is no such thing as me getting "a little sick." *Please let this be allergies*. No such luck. I spent the next couple of days lying flat on my back and drinking plenty of fluids. As usual, Joan was a gem of a neighbor, coming over three times a day to take Sadie out for a walk.

The last time I was sick like this, I was worried that Dave would catch it from me. He didn't, but it was nice having someone here to care that I was sick, to at least *know* I was sick. Besides the fact that I'm feeling brain-dead from watching eight hours of television today, I feel so alone. I've always been a self-described "island." You'd never know it considering how social I appear, but the truth is, I've generally been very happy being on my own. That's how I grew up and how it was for a very long time. I counted on me and no one else, at least until I married Dave. But even after Dave and I married, I was still comfortable doing things alone.

Only a few months after the wedding, I announced that I wanted to learn Spanish. I inquired about the tuition of a nearby language school and discovered I could spend a month in Mexico on the Baja California Peninsula at an immersion college where I could learn the language for the same cost as the local school. With Dave's persuasive writing skills, he wrote a letter to my employer asking them to give me a month of vacation time. I wasn't asking for reimbursement of the costs, just for the time off. It worked like a charm, and we timed the whole trip so Dave and I could visit midway when he came out to California on a business thing. And after we retired, a couple of times a year I'd spend a few days camping with the dog. It was great for both of us.

So I've never had a problem being alone. But now it's different. When you have someone who loves you to the moon and back, being physically alone is not the same as being lonely. But when you don't have that someone anymore, when you don't have that witness to your life, being alone takes on a whole new dimension.

The other day, while on my back nursing myself to health, I spent as much time online as I did in front of the television.

I stumbled on a weird psychological study done back in the 1950s. A doctor named Curt Richter, a professor at Johns Hopkins, did an experiment with rats. I'm certainly not trying to promote using animals in the laboratory; I abhor animal testing! But it happened, and the results are interesting. Without going into all the variables of the experiment, the gist is that Dr. Richter wanted to expand on a study by Walter Cannon, the man who coined the phrase "fight or flight." Cannon's 1942 research was on "voodoo death," or essentially being scared to death. Richter wanted to answer the question whether fear can actually cause death.

To research the theory of voodoo death, Dr. Richter took several rats, some domesticated and some wild, and dropped them into buckets of water to see how long they could swim before they drowned. I know, repulsive and cruel, right? He found the majority of them lasted less than fifteen minutes. However, he also found that if they were pulled out of the water right before they drowned, then dried off, held for a bit, and allowed to recover, they could swim for sixty hours! Those poor rats swam for sixty hours simply because they had *hope*—hope that someone was going to reach their hand into the water any minute and save them. Of course, science experiments often being cruel, they were all allowed to drown. Sickening.

The takeaway here is that hope affects your life. Studies show that within six months of a cancer diagnosis, the risk of heart attack or stroke is more than twice that seen in people without cancer.[4] If you read PubMed, something that has come quite naturally to me since Dave's cancer diagnosis, they give many physical reasons for that. But isn't there a chance that the real reason people have a heart attack within the first six months is that some of them consider a cancer diagnosis to be a death sentence? They give up all hope and are afraid. Could the real reason the risk of heart attack and stroke increases be that they're scared to death? Now, I'm not talking about several years down the road; after all the treatments that are in a cancer patient's path, it seems obvious that the body would be subject to a greater threat of other maladies. But I'm concerned only with the early stages.

It's fourteen months after Dave's diagnosis. Dave has undergone all the surgeries he will ever have. Five days earlier, he was diagnosed with his second recurrence of squamous cell carcinoma. Historically, the statistics are very bad for him.

Dr. Thorn calls me one morning to discuss the medical plan. We spend nearly forty-five minutes on the phone; I take detailed notes the entire time. Eventually, I put all the information in an email to Dave, partially for his knowledge and partially so I can document this phone call. I make nearly a dozen bullet points, highlighting the good and the not-so-good. I finish my email with these paragraphs:

> I told him all about the plant-based diet, alkaline water, beetroot powder, amla powder, etc. I said if it's helped one hundred people it's well worth trying. He believes 100% our positive attitude, yet not sticking our heads in the sand, is crucial, and he said if there's a 1% chance of a diet working he would do it too.

> I spoke to him about stages and life expectancy. I read a very scary article and needed to know his thoughts. I don't think that's stuff you want to know, so I won't share. If you do, let me know. But speaking to him gave me more hope than I had before. I

complimented him up the ying yang for his patience and understanding and availability. He's the kindest surgeon I have ever known.

Thorn will email Shilo tonight to let him know I am now in the loop, and as soon as everything is coordinated at the hospital they will be in touch. The tumor board is just a formality. I think if there was going to be surgery, they would have to wait for the board.

I hope you have an absolutely great day! This is really terrific news! You really are a BEAST! And we're gonna have a flipping awesome time in this new camper. :-)

I love you!

Months after that email, Dave and I are at the university hospital finishing up an appointment with Dr. Shilo when Dave asks me to leave the room. For real? Yes, Dave would like a minute alone with our oncologist.

Snoop Dog has much difficulty not hovering near the closed door where Dave and Dr. Shilo converse, but out of respect for Dave I manage to stay on the other side of the hallway. Yes, there is a burning curiosity inside me, and Dave knows it.

On the three-hour drive home, he chuckles as I nonchalantly pry about the subject of their conversation before I finally drop it.

Months later, Dave and I are sitting on the deck of our favorite coffee shop. It's a beautiful day. Out of the blue, Dave decides to tell me what he and Dr. Shilo had discussed that day behind the closed door.

Dave had asked the doctor how he would die from this cancer. Will it be painful? Will it be a long, drawn-out death? Dr. Shilo said Dave is more likely to die from complications such as a heart attack, stroke, or brain bleed.

I think back to how I was preparing for a death that wouldn't come as a surprise, a death that would probably follow hospice care. This new information suggests to me that it may be a surprise after all, and I'm not sure I'm happy about that. This means I may wake up one morning to find Dave no longer alive beside me.

Looking back on those conversations with our doctors, I'm reminded that Dave and I were never afraid . . . and there was always *hope*. Dave still had hope right up to the love letter that he wrote me two months ago. He said besides being a difficult letter to write, he didn't finish it because he never gave up. And neither did I. Even when death was predicted to be two to three weeks down the road, Dave and I continued our days like that number was not set in stone. And it wasn't. Dave lived just shy of six more weeks.

Except for my momentary meltdowns, we dealt with his cancer without fear, and we always had hope. But what about now?

Now that I feel forlorn, lost, and alone?

Now that I don't have my person to give me silent confidence?

Now that I don't have someone I love driving that hope?

Now that hope for *my* life is different from what it was for *our* lives?

It's no surprise that I can reduce the *quality* of my life by remaining in constant sadness, but is it possible that I can actually reduce my lifespan as well? If I continue to follow a healthy diet, participate in regular physical activity, and get my medical checkups, is it possible I will still actually shorten my life by having an ominous mindset?

And is this possibly the reason faith in something or someone greater than ourselves leads to hope? A simple Google search shows that faith and hope are intimately connected. Although my gut tells me faith comes first and then leads to hope, my reading suggests otherwise. It suggests that hope is a wish for a desired outcome: I hope the surgery is successful . . . I hope the sun is shining tomorrow . . . I hope I get to spend the rest of my life with Dave.

Faith is much stronger. Faith is a strong belief in something you cannot see or prove: I have faith the surgery will be successful . . . I have faith the sun will be shining tomorrow, so I'm planning a picnic . . . I have faith I will get to spend the rest of my life with Dave.

I don't think that faith has to be spiritual, although I believe that's the usual connotation. If I say, "I have a strong faith," the listener may believe I'm saying I have a strong belief in God. But if I say, "I have faith that the rain will stop before my basement floods," does that have anything to do with God? Or am I really saying that I hope with all my heart the rain stops, in which case I'd define faith as wishful thinking?

This seems to be a rabbit hole I've wandered down, and my black-and-white-thinking brain will once again not receive any concrete answers. However, Cathy turned me on to the television series *The Chosen.* It's probably something I never would have watched six months or six years ago, but things change. Needs change. Being that I was sick on the couch, I decided to binge-watch the first season. I like it! I think it's so much easier to follow the Bible stories by watching rather than reading. I find it interesting that I get extremely emotional when "a God event" occurs on the show. It doesn't even have to be a miracle, just something that supports the notion of faith. I wonder whether there's any connection between these tears and the tears that always fall when I pray or when I'm in church. Furthermore, is there any connection between those tears and the ones that come when I speak to Mandy and I touch upon a truth deep within me? This is all very thought-provoking.

Today, Megan reached out to me with a heart emoji. We've barely spoken since Dave died. I'm sure she misses her father, and I suppose she misses me too. Then Patrick's boys called to thank me for their Christmas cards—and the check that came inside each one. They both said "love you" when they hung up the phone.

Did this all happen today as a result of a budding faith within me?

Even an island needs an occasional visitor.

39

Friday, December 15

I've had a few really rough days. Being sick has been no picnic, but fortunately, for the first time in forever, this head cold looks like it's not going to become a sinus infection followed by bronchitis, which I'm thrilled about.

Physically I'm feeling better than earlier in the week, but emotionally I'm a train wreck. You know that game "Six Degrees of Kevin Bacon" where every actor can be connected to Kevin Bacon by no more than six people? I feel like I'm living the game of "Two Degrees of Dave Gilbride." Everything I look at, everything I touch, everything I hear reminds me of Dave. No matter how remote and disconnected to Dave it is, it connects me to a memory of him.

I think about him constantly: the early days when we were first married and I didn't know how lucky I was; the later days, yet still before cancer, when I felt like we were the luckiest people in the world; and the cancer days, when we lived our lives to the fullest while trying to beat cancer, or at least manage it. And then there were the final days, the ones I still can't wrap my head around, the ones when I was focused on the task of managing a pain-free death and feel I somehow forgot in the process that he would actually be dead at the end of it all.

One of Dave's jobs around the house was going through the mail. Back in the day when we both worked, Dave had very few domestic chores, but since retirement I gave him some stuff to do. Sorting the mail was one of those chores. He actually liked going through the mail. Changing the filters for the HVAC system and rolling out the garbage cans to the street were two others. Of course, I would gladly have done any of these, but once Dave retired from the town manager position due to cancer, his days became a lot longer with a lot less to fill them up. So, I would call these chores "Penis Jobs." This concept came from my mother, whose mindset for some things is stuck in the '50s and '60s when she grew up: "You need a penis to do the job." Not literally, of course, and she never actually said that, but it meant it was a job for a man. Dave always laughed when I'd come up with something for him to do and tell him it was a penis job. He knew there was no getting out of it.

Anyway, most of the mail is crap. Like most people nowadays, I do everything online. Yesterday there was one piece of mail. It was from Medicare. I knew immediately what it was. I knew because I've been taking care of anything related to our medical insurance since Dave and I got married. When Dave turned sixty-five, we registered him for Medicare. My medical insurance, a benefit from retiring from my cop job, became Dave's secondary insurance, which covered the remaining 20 percent that Medicare didn't. Oh, how many times we thanked our lucky stars that we had that insurance! Dave used to tease me that he married me for my pension and my medical benefits. Well, if he knew how useful that insurance would be twenty years after we married, he wouldn't have been just teasing; we racked up somewhere in the vicinity of $2.5 million in medical bills but never paid more than around $300, if that.

Since the cancer, I've stayed on top of all the billing by checking the Medicare and private insurance websites frequently so I can jump on any potential issues before they become problems. That's how my brain works—constantly searching for something to fix . . . an OCD thing. Sometime after Dave died, out of curiosity, I attempted to pull up the Medicare site to see what hospice had cost the government for the month of October. I was denied access. Clearly when it had been reported to Social Security that Dave was deceased, not only did his Social Security account become inaccessible, but his Medicare account did as well. So the nice folks decided to send me a paper statement in the mail. There's never more than a moment to escape thoughts of Dave.

I really can't understand why I find all this so difficult to comprehend. I'm a smart woman with realistic expectations. Even though I never focused on Dave dying, I knew it was going to happen, so why can't I believe this is real? Why do I find it so unfathomable that I will never see him again . . . never talk to him again? I remind myself he's no longer in pain, just as he reminded me when we discussed my fear of dying. But it's just not enough. And I'm finding it downright scary that this may never feel any different.

Generally, I'm not afraid of much. Okay, actually? The truth? Thirty-five years ago I entered the hiring process for my cop job. Part of the process was completing a psychological exam that consisted of a written exam and an interview. I could see in the written exam they were looking for consistency and trying to weed out the people who might want this job for the wrong reasons. It doesn't take a brain surgeon to figure that out.

I remember in the interview, the doctor asked me what I was afraid of. Well, I knew my number-one fear was my own death; it always has been since I was a little girl. But some how I thought that wouldn't be an ideal answer considering I was applying for a law enforcement position. So my twenty-four-year-old self instead gave him my number two fear: fear of failure. That was the absolute truth! Being a perfectionist like I am, failure doesn't bode well with me. Over the years, those fears have changed. Once cancer came around, fear of my death became overshadowed by fear of Dave's death. Isn't it far worse to lose the one you love than your own life?

With the exception of caring for Dave, I kicked my fear of failure a long time ago. There was no room for error there. Maybe "kicked" is a strong word, but I'm much gentler with myself. Now I believe in trying until you get it right. All those marvelous quotes about failure applying only to quitters helped me tremendously because, if I have nothing else, I have tenacity. As a matter of fact, Dave and I visited Cooperstown, New York, this past July. I have a picture of me pointing at a sign that read, "It's hard to beat a person who never gives up," courtesy of Babe Ruth. That certainly applied to Dave and me! Once Dave died, I had no more fear. Absolutely nothing. Heights, spiders, snakes, dark alleys, getting in a fight . . . nope, no fear.

But I do fear being this sad for the rest of my life. I fear not taking joy in the days anymore. I fear my days remaining colorless. I fear waking up every day at 7 a.m. only to think that in fourteen hours I can go back to bed. And I truly fear living another twenty years of sadness only to look back and regret how I wasted the last twenty years of my life.

It kind of feels like being at the bottom of a forty-foot well where I'm able to do all the normal, daily tasks. Friends periodically call, text, or stick their heads over the side of the well and shout down, "How you holding up, Patty?"

I respond with, "Doing the best I can!"

"Let me know if there's anything I can do," they shout as they go about their day while I sit at the bottom of the well. Occasionally I have enough distractions that I'm lifted a foot off the bottom, but I'm still thirty-nine feet down. And when those distractions are over, I'm right back at a forty-foot drop.

I feel completely abnormal . . . peculiar . . . downright fucked up. For someone who has had the overwhelming majority of her life under control—minus the cancer—it's absolutely terrifying.

Today's big fail was in something as simple as deciding to wash my sheets. Sometime over the last month, I washed and folded the bright-blue sheet and the yellow pillowcase Dave last used. We had a buttercup-yellow fitted sheet on our bed, but when Dave started having accidents, I replaced it with a dark-gray sheet. Today I thought I'd return the dark-gray sheet to the linen closet and make the bed with the yellow one. After I stretched it out, I saw that the stains didn't come out the last time I washed it. They're still there, and they brought back every memory of how those stains got there. I threw the sheet in the garbage.

40

Sunday, December 17

*T*oday is week seven. One week from today will be Christmas Eve. I don't expect I'll feel a whole lot different, or even a little different, in another week.

For many years now, people have told me how strong I am, often saying, "You're one of the strongest women I know." Dave even mentioned during one of our Tub Talks how I can be a little "intimidating" to his kids and to be aware of that when he's no longer able to be a communication buffer. He suggested I remember WWDD when crossing difficult paths with them. I feel a little guilty that although I listened to what he said, I didn't feel a tremendous amount of compassion. Dave's kids are all incredibly smart, well-educated people in their forties. Granted, they had a mother who had severe mental health issues, but they were raised by their dad for most of their young lives. And their dad, although certainly not the perfect father, was always an amazing source of support and strength from the beginning of fatherhood to the day he died . . . seven weeks ago today.

I never had a rock of support like that when I was a kid. My parents divorced when I was four years old. Although I was the apple of my alcoholic father's eye, naturally he wasn't able to provide a safe, secure environment. Not to mention I lost him when I was only ten. Being that my mother was a young woman when they divorced, she was actively dating for most of my childhood. I was probably about thirty years old when I finally told her about that sexual trauma that occurred at the hands of her boyfriend when I was just a child. I never thought it mattered. I never believed that someone taking away my ability to say no at that early age would have an effect on me for the rest of my life.

I started making lots of bad choices regarding boys in my teen years. By the time I was seventeen, those choices left me with a broken nose. I went to college for a year and then dropped out. My mother had moved to Virginia with her boyfriend while I was away at school. I moved in with them only for a couple of months until I found a place of my own and a way to support myself. My entire life, I never knew someone I could borrow twenty bucks from—until Dave.

Before I met Dave, I was solely responsible for building my productive life. After bouncing around for a handful of years, still making bad choices in relationships, I entered the hiring process for my civil service job with the sheriff's department. It took over a year to get hired, but eventually I did. I was twenty-five years old when I entered the police academy and couldn't have guessed in a million years what a smart move that was.

By the time I was thirty, I'd saved enough money to buy a house. I loved it! My house and my dogs were everything to me. I was so poor that I learned how to fix everything myself, and this was before YouTube. The only person I was ever able to consistently count on was me. I enjoyed my job and was good at it. I could think on my feet. And as the years went on, my confidence increased because I made smart decisions at work and became handy around the house.

I didn't date often, and when I did I dated from the same mold my mother had: someone who would lead me to heartache, someone who cared more about himself than his partner.

This was around the time I first started serving legal papers to Dave at work.

After a few years of social conversation during these visits to his office was when Dave started to drop those hints about seeing each other outside of work, even if it was only to watch Megan play at a soccer game. Although his sense of humor and friendly nature were the first things to catch my attention, I always passed on his invitations because he lacked that "bad boy" gene. I imagine from Dave's perspective he saw an attractive woman in her mid-thirties who had a responsible job and financial independence, was easy to talk to, and appeared to really have her shit together. But he had no idea how broken I was inside.

A couple of years later were the trips to Hawaii and Jamaica. What started out as snookering an invite on a company incentive trip because I wanted a break from the New Jersey winter turned into something I never would have imagined. It was because Dave was such a caring gentleman on the Hawaii trip that I became charmed and stupefied that someone would be so kind without an ulterior motive. It was because he made me feel like I was the most important person in the room that I started to say to myself, "Maybe it's time to make a change. This bad boy thing hasn't been working so well for you, Patty."

When we spent that one week in Hawaii, I was a captive audience to Dave's pure goodness. At that time in my life, it had never once occurred to me that I just might deserve pure goodness. So by the time Jamaica rolled around a couple of weeks later, I was thinking of Dave in a slightly different light. That afternoon on the balcony of the Ritz-Carlton while sharing a lounge chair and a bottle of Mad Annie's rum sealed the deal. Talking for hours, being physically close with no threat of anything more unless it was my decision, gave me the safe, secure environment I needed to fall in love. This is why by the time we came home from the trip I was fairly confident Dave was the man I would marry.

If I had to give our marriage a score on a scale of 1–10, I'd give the first dozen years before we retired a solid 7. We all have our own garbage we bring into a relationship, and there's always stuff that could be improved on, yet we don't often take the time to get at the root and work on things.

After we retired and all our garbage came to a head, we went through that five-month separation. Dave and I never stopped loving each other during that time; we just needed to figure out if we really wanted to be together and, if so, how to make it better. By the time he moved back into the house, we'd started to work on the important things. Clearly, I had a whole lot of garbage stemming from the time I was seven years old that needed to be dealt with. Dave was there and supported me every step of the way. This was when our relationship became a 9. A nine is pretty damned good if you ask me! Loving, trusting, honest, safe, fun, and with a complete respect for one another's amazing qualities along with an acceptance of one another's flaws, is how I describe our relationship for the five years that followed, but before cancer.

Cancer is a "make it or break it" test for a marriage. Oddly enough, a part of Dave was always surprised at how much I stuck to him like a magnet after his diagnosis. This is an excerpt from his last love letter to me:

> Knowing what a burden I was going to become over these last few years I suppose I fully expected you to run like hell and leave me to the whims of social services or something. You didn't. Your relentless pursuit of my treatments, my nutrition, my comfort, etc. . . . and willingness to let slide some of my little tantrums and outbursts have been a marvel. You are a "force of nature" and a person to be reckoned with.

Knowing that your efforts are all coming from a place of love, I am particularly saddened when I see you cry, or hold back tears, and it is clear that the stress of all of this is taking a toll on you. I wish that when the dust settles you could hop a flight to Aruba, first class, and stay in a fancy hotel with beach access and great restaurants, and recharge your batteries. Give it some thought, OK?

Fighting for Dave's life during cancer? Well, that brought our marriage to an 11. Yep, skipped right past 10. Ten is what happens when you love and trust each other completely, when you would die for one another. Eleven is when you find something more than love . . . something undefinable . . .

If past behavior is an indication of future behavior, and if my life has been essentially a success story, I believe I should have the confidence that I *will* come out the other end of this even stronger than before. By the time I started to share my life with Dave, I'd done pretty well for myself considering where I came from. Thanks to Dave's enduring love, and to visits to a great therapist, the rest of me healed as well. It would be such a waste to have done so much healing only to crumble when the one who helped heal me is no longer here.

41

Tuesday, December 19

*Y*esterday I saw Mandy. I have so much to talk to her about every time I see her. My thoughts are disorganized and I don't know where to start. I'm one of those therapy patients who usually walk in with a mental outline of what they intend to cover during each session. Mandy is used to that. But I'm unable to form those outlines these days.

We spoke quite a bit about my relationship with Megan. Moving forward, I believe this will be one of the most important relationships I have. We talked about how I never knew what a good father could be until I met Dave and his kids. The way he supported them, didn't interfere in their decisions, always had money when they were in need . . . I can't imagine being a girl with a dad like that. How do some people get so lucky? Is that actually the norm?

After my session, I reached out to Megan and we chatted for about twenty minutes. I'm amazed by how well-adjusted she sounds since her father's death. I understand she has much more to keep her busy than I do, and she may be showing only her best side so as not to burden me. I hope she's doing as well as she sounds, but I'm rather jealous that she's getting along better than me. I'm also perturbed at myself for being jealous. When we speak, I don't hide my grief from her, nor do I appear strong. Most people haven't seen me let down all my walls, so this is definitely the start of something new.

I told Megan I believe she's going to be an important part of my healing. She said she would be honored to help. I reminded her that each of us is the closest thing to Dave the other one has, and as much as I absolutely hate to admit it, now that Dave has died, my only fear now is getting old and needing someone—physically needing someone. It actually turns my stomach to think of being dependent on someone other than my husband. But that's the reality. I imagine I wouldn't be so concerned with this if I had my own kids to handle this obligation, but Dave's kids are the closest thing I have.

I wasted some time this afternoon watching short reels on Facebook. There was one called "Every stranger has a story." This guy walks up to someone and asks a thought-provoking question. The question he asked today to a woman who was walking her dog was, "Who was your greatest love, and why did you fall in love with them?" Of course I was hooked with that question. The woman said that Bill, her husband of forty-one years, was her greatest love, and she just lost him. Now I was really hooked.

She smiled when she told the story of how they met, much the same way Dave and I used to smile and laugh when we told our story to people. Bill was her best friend and had the best sense of humor; I sat there nodding my head. They giggled for forty-one years; Dave's humor was a bit more intellectual than giggle-worthy. Generally, I was responsible for the laughter that resulted in giggles, but I appreciate the similarities her love shares with mine.

And then, as though it were me talking instead of her, she said, "His eyes smiled. He had really twinkly eyes that smiled at you, and I miss that so much. I was so in love with this man. I just wanted to be with him all the time. I can't even say he was a partner; we were one. I wouldn't be the same human being without him. I don't feel he left me; I feel he just went ahead of me." I was so impressed with that last sentence. What a healthy way to feel!

At the end, the interviewer asked the woman for her name. "Patty," she replied. What are the chances of that? She finished the interview saying she was so appreciative of the question and the walk down memory lane.

Somehow, other women out in the world have lost the love of their lives and are managing to continue living. This has to get easier for me. It just has to.

Thursday, December 21

I've been a mess these last two days. An absolute train wreck. So yesterday when my friend Chris-from-the-beach invited me to be her plus one for a spiritual reading webinar, I said, "Sure! What have I got to lose?" The medium was offering a buy one, get one. Being that Chris hopes to connect with not only her recently departed husband but her son who passed several years before, she has done a few of these readings.

As I went about the day, I reached out to Dave several times to remind him of solid signs he could convey to the medium should he be able to show up. I know he doesn't interrupt others and is sensitive to their needs, but I figured if there were a slew of spirits milling about waiting to connect with this medium, I'd need Dave to bust in there like there's a Morton's steak and a bowl of homemade vanilla ice cream waiting for him. And although Dave should know the signs I consider solid, because we've discussed them—in life and in death—I didn't want to take any chances he'd forget.

Anyway, the reading last night was uneventful. There were about thirty-five attendees and two mediums. One of the mediums was clear, quiet, reserved . . . believable. The other was . . . a loose cannon, even a bit annoying. It's possible

Chris's son reached out, as the loose cannon was connecting to two sons at the same time. Eh. It all seemed sketchy and unauthentic to me. And I wasn't disappointed that Dave didn't show up. I still don't know whether I believe in all this spirit stuff. If he's out there, I'm certain he will find a way to comfort me. Love like this doesn't die.

This morning I had an appointment at the county courthouse to probate the will. My appointment was about ten minutes from where my mother lives. I thought about calling her and telling her I'd stop by when I was done, but why? To talk? Our conversations so often go south, even when we're trying to be on our best behavior. I'm still extremely angry at some things she said around the time of Dave's death. I doubt I'll ever forgive her. At the very least, I don't have the emotional bandwidth for her. She sucks the life out of me, and I need whatever energy I do have to deal with my own life right now.

As I walked up the ramp to the courthouse, my phone rang. It was my mother. She rarely calls me, so I figured it was important. Turns out her annual rent increase came through and she's having some issues with the office. Although we have a broken relationship, I do handle all her financial matters. We spoke for only five minutes, yet in that short time she managed to make me crazy. I told her I'd come to her apartment when I was done at the courthouse.

Seated in the hallway of the "wills and probate court," I quietly waited for my name to be called. I whispered to myself that I had the strength to muddle through this: *Put on your business face, handle the task, and set aside your tears. You have the rest of the day to cry.*

Tina, the deputy clerk, called my name and we proceeded to her office. She had Christmas decorations scattered about, and it reminded me of how the clerical staff in the sheriff's department used to decorate the office I worked in.

It didn't take long for tears to leak out. I believe it was her second question that primed them: "And your relationship to the decedent?"

"He was my husband," I said.

She offered her condolences, and I was thankful she was much nicer than the person I'd spoken to on the phone.

Tina read through all the forms I filled out as well as Dave's Last Will and Testament, and she had a couple more forms for me to complete. While I filled in the blanks, she told me her dad died two and a half years ago. She said her mom says she's okay, but Tina knows she's not. I said, "You're right. She's not."

Tina can't visit her mom this Christmas, but her brother lives nearby, so her mom won't be alone. I was surprised to hear her mom lives near Hazleton, Pennsylvania. I remembered the year I dragged Megan and Dave to Hazleton, which is full of mountains, for an organized bike ride. As usual, Megan and I rode at our pace while Dave rode at his more leisurely pace behind us, smelling the roses. The best part of finishing those rides was finding the nearest diner afterward and eating everything in sight, something all three of us did well!

I snapped back to the present when Tina said, "They say it gets better after a year, but it doesn't really. You just find a way to manage."

I know what she said is true.

It was because of the death of her father that Tina took this job. She wanted to be able to help other people during a difficult time while also keeping his memory alive. He loved photography, and she pointed to the large, framed prints on the wall.

"He liked lighthouses?" I asked.

She named all the lighthouses she'd brought her dad to visit when he came to North Carolina to see her. I completely understood wanting to keep his memory alive. It's so important to me to keep Dave's memory alive.

I wonder whether I'll have enough of an impact on those I love so they try to keep my memory alive. Or is it just this important to me because I'm completely neurotic when it comes to all things related to death and dying?

I finished up. The will was probated. Tina handed me a pile of papers and a receipt for the $30 cash, and Dave's life is now all wrapped up. It sounds so benign.

Begrudgingly, I headed over to my mother's apartment, picking up a coffee and getting out some more tears on the way over. We talked for over an hour about Dave and how I feel without him. She's hurting too. She very carefully filtered her words to avoid an ugly scene; apparently she can do it when it's important to her. I generally don't talk to my mother about anything personal, but I don't even consider my grief to be a personal matter anymore. I've been such a private person for so many years, and now I don't have the slightest concern about sharing this immense vulnerability.

By the time I arrived home, it was later than usual. Sadie and I headed to the beach for a walk. Today is the winter solstice. Even though I'm no fan of winter, I like this day because it means after today the days will get longer. By the time we returned home, it was time for dinner and my daily shot of rock and bourbon.

While I was eating dinner, Jeremy called. Since I just spoke to him a couple of days ago, it seemed odd for him to check in again. But that's what he was doing . . . just checking in. This is definitely an area of life that Jeremy is not comfortable with, but he really held his own. Probably because I blubbered in his ear, he said he'd been wondering how long it would take for me to completely break down. I told him he has no idea how much breaking down I've been doing when no one is around.

"You've been an absolute rock for your entire life," he shared. "Now it's time for you to cry." I then told him I feel like a completely useless, weak, waste of life, to which he astutely said, "That's how you're supposed to feel right now."

I told Jeremy it's been almost eight weeks now since Dave died, and I'm still questioning whether I said everything I needed to say to him. Since we knew he was going to die, I had time that many people don't have. And being that my brain never stops moving, I was sure I'd thought of and shared every question . . . every topic . . . every memory so that I would have no regrets after Dave was gone. But I wasn't prepared for so many earlier memories of Dave to run through my head so often. That was a time when Dave loved me just a little more than I loved him. I never really gave it any thought. But now I'm thinking of those early days and feeling guilty that I didn't love him as much as he deserved. Did I tell Dave any of this? Did he know that he completely changed my life . . . that he made me the person I am today . . . that his love changed me for the better?

It's amazing that Jeremy could understand a word I said as I cried and shared all these fears with him. At one point he stated, "Now that's the one thing I'm not going to let you say. Dave and I talked about our wives, the effect they've had on our lives, and there wasn't a doubt in Dave's mind that he knew how important each of you were to each other. You can cry all you want. I'm okay with that. But don't you doubt for a minute that Dave didn't know just how you felt about him."

As we got off the phone, FedEx rapped on the door to let me know they dropped a package on the front steps. When I spoke to Megan the other day, she told me she sent a Christmas present. I told her I believe I'm the hardest person in the world to buy for, that she didn't have to send me presents, and that I still carry a lot of leftover issues from the overabundance of gifts my mother gave me. She replied, "I think you'll like it."

I ripped through all the packaging and saw the most perfect Christmas present anyone could have given me: a pretty beaded bracelet personalized with the letters WWDD. I had just stopped crying from Jeremy's call and the waterworks turned on again. I texted her immediately to tell her it was perfect! Unbeknownst to me, these "little words" bracelets are all the rage now. She couldn't have nailed it any better.

As I blubbered, this time via text, to the third person in one day about what a completely weak, useless, sloppy mess I am, Megan replied with, "Maybe that's good for you. Like you've always been the useful, put together, least mess of a person I know. Maybe this is letting you take a break but you just can't see that right now."

I told her I worry that my "strong, confident self" went out the window and wonder how that happened so fast. I don't "do vulnerable well." She suggested it hasn't gone out the window but is just sitting on a bookshelf for the time being.

After we said our goodbyes, I headed for a hot shower and thought, *I can't believe I cried to three people today. There was a time when I never cried in front of anyone. Over the years I learned to cry in front of Dave. And now? Three people in one day!* I shook my head.

Then I did what I have done in every hot shower I have taken since Dave died: After the shower door steams up, using my finger I write the words "Dave, I love you" followed by a heart and an infinity sign. I squeegeed it away five minutes later.

42

Friday, December 22

Dave is shaving while I chatter about two houses I've looked at. "The realtor says the owner is moving the master bed and bath to the back of the house, so I want to look at that one again," I tell him. He nods while he looks in the mirror and continues shaving. I decide I should ask him to come look at the houses. There are always things guys look at that women don't see, and besides, two pairs of eyes are better than one.

But I know he's not coming to live in this house with me. Why isn't he coming with me? He's not going to Florida again. Oh, wait. I know. It's because he's dead.

As that thought comes through my mind, I feel my body being sucked from dreamland into consciousness.

I lay there in the dark digesting this dream. My great-great-grandmother's clock chimed four times as I absorbed the immensity of the dream and started to cry. I cried not only over the dream and because Dave is dead, but I cried because I don't have him here to comfort me after a bad dream.

Some people believe that when we dream of the departed, it's really their spirit visiting us because this is the only time most of us have cleared our minds enough that we can accept such a subtle visitor from the other side. I don't believe that, but I hedged my bet; I reached up to the ceiling and said out loud, "Thanks for visiting, Hon, but that was really, really difficult."

Lying in bed, I heard Sadie's gentle snoring stop. My crying woke her up. I heard one chime from the clock and realized I'd been contemplating this dream for a full half hour. Still not settling back into sleep, I eventually heard five chimes as I started to drift.

Sunday, December 24

I woke this morning to another dream of Dave. Although some believe that dreams can be visits from your dearly departed, spirit mediums will also tell you that not all dreams are visits. If they make you cry, they're not visits, but if you feel like you've been wrapped in a warm hug, that's a visit.

What I find odd is that this was the second dream in the last few days in which I realize Dave is gone while I'm still in the dream.

> *I'm on my way to assist my fellow officers in a raid this evening, and Dave is joining me. He's driving our car, I'm in the passenger seat, and we're in the town he worked in when we first met. He's angry and hot-tempered for some reason. He drops me off in town and goes home. Not knowing the time of the raid, I walk to the meeting location and text one of the guys running the job.*

> *Night has suddenly fallen, but it's too early for the raid to start. It's only around 7 p.m., and we usually muster for these events about 2 a.m. There's a car parked across the street from the building I walked to, and I can see a light in it. It's the light from the screen of the person I just texted*

as he replies to me saying we may as well meet now since everyone is here.

We're in the building, and I need to let Dave know he doesn't need to come. I'm afraid I will hurt his feelings, as he was looking forward to doing this. I try to call him on my cell phone and have constant difficulties. I can't dial the number; the icons keep jumping around, and my contacts are all messed up. I pull out my laptop, which I suddenly have, as well as my tablet. Eventually I'm able to call him and tell him the group will not need him to join. I tell him he should rest anyway because he sounds like he's getting a cold.

Just when I hang up the phone, I realize I should have told him what we have in the fridge for him to eat. I just bought English muffins, and if he toasts one he could make a PB&J and the peanut butter will get all gooey. But, I think, that won't matter to him since he can't taste food anymore.

Suddenly, I visualize that Dave no longer has a nose. When we were in the car, he had a nose as well as the extra weight he used to carry around. As I'm sitting around a conference table with all my fellow officers, I suddenly remember Dave is dead.

Who was I talking to? What just happened there?

I put my face in my hands and tell the team leader, "You're not going to believe this, but that call to my husband . . . he died last week." The team leader lets out a spontaneous laugh and pushes away from the table as he stands and walks away. The rest of the team just looks at me as we arrange ourselves in groups for the raid. I lie on the floor with my pad and pencil, ready to take notes, thinking about what just happened and how I'm going to get used to Dave being dead.

I woke from the dream, and before my eyes were even open I wondered what time it was. I couldn't believe this happened again. I fluttered my eyes open a crack to see if there was any light in the room. I took a guess that it was about 6:30 a.m. as I reached over to check the time. Sure enough, it was 6:37. No need to go back to sleep. But I knew it was going to be a long day if it started this early. As I rolled back to Dave's side of the bed, I whispered, "Dave, it's Christmas Eve. I love you and I miss you."

Christmas Eve . . . one of the dreaded "firsts." Based on when Dave died, the last "first" will be our wedding anniversary on September 7. Yes, that will be much more difficult than Christmas because the whole day revolved around the two of us making a commitment to spend our lives honoring each other. Not to mention, we had an absolute blast at our wedding! It was the perfect day!

Besides all the Christmas memories being painful, another awful aspect to deal with this time of year is that everyone is so damned happy! Everything around me is a celebration of Christmas: music, decorations, hustle and bustle in the stores, wishes from everyone of Merry Christmas and Happy New Year . . . Can I just bury my head in the sand?

Christmas is a mixed bag of emotions for me. As a young child, I had the typical excitement about the holiday. My parents separated when I was three years old, and my mother and I moved to an apartment. My mom did a nice job decorating our apartment and setting up the artificial tree. There were always special ornaments that were handed down from her mother placed in a position of prominence on the tree.

Being that I was so young at the time, a friend's mother would watch me after nursery school while my mother worked. She was a nice German lady, but she felt it was important for me to know the real story about St. Nicholas, thereby telling me, "Santa Claus doesn't exist" when I was only four years old. Yes, I dealt with reality at a very early age. I kept this secret from my mother for many years. I remember wondering how long I could let her think I believed in Santa. One year, when I was about six or seven, I actually looked out my bedroom window because I thought I heard Santa landing on the roof. It's amazing what you can believe in with a little faith.

For as long as I can remember, my mother always bought me an obscene amount of presents that we couldn't afford. I'd start opening presents at around 9 a.m. and still be at it five or more hours later. We would even break for lunch! This continued for decades. The unfortunate part is that I knew we couldn't afford these presents, and to be honest, the whole process was actually very boring. After opening each present and saying, "oooh . . . aaahhhh . . . just what I wanted," I'd be making a mental note whether this was one of the presents that would go back to the store. My mother didn't care what I kept and what I returned. The next day, we'd spend the entire day returning twenty or thirty presents, then all the cash from those presents would provide me with a "credit" to buy something else. It was a very strange way to grow up, and I had absolutely no control of the situation.

My mom did this because shopping made *her* feel good, not because it made *me* feel good. Every Christmas she continued to shop in the same fashion. For decades, no matter how much I pleaded with her to stop, she wouldn't. I was twenty-five when I started my career, and by the time I was thirty I'd bought my house. Even though I spent every dollar I had on the house and there were many things I wanted and couldn't afford, I dreaded Christmas because of my mother's uncontrollable gift buying.

After decades of this, I despised opening presents, not just from her but from anyone. All it represented was having absolutely no control and needing to decide what I was going to have to give up. One year I had an all-out crying fit when I told my mother she must stop doing this. Her reply was, "I can't believe you are taking away this one thing that makes me happy." She thought I was being selfish! I'm still baffled that she said that. For decades she made me unhappy on Christmas. How could that make a mother happy?

Sometime after I bought my house, she asked if she could wrap and keep presents in my finished basement. Since she lived in a tiny studio apartment, I said she could, but with the warning to control her buying. That year was the straw that broke the camel's back. I went into the basement one day and saw a bedsheet covering the presents. I hadn't realized how quickly the stash had become a massive pile. I lifted the sheet and saw at least forty presents, and they were all wrapped. I called my mom and told her to come to my house. When she arrived, I said she needed to pick out ten presents and those would be the ten she would give me on Christmas Day. The rest she could take home, unwrap, and return to the store. I told her that this year *she* would be the one to decide what to keep and what to return; this year *she* would be the one to spend all day making returns. Of course she was angry, and I ended up lying on my bed, crying for hours.

It certainly wouldn't have taken a psychology major to look at my childhood—divorce, father dying, sexual trauma, my mother's inability to hear my wishes—and figure that OCD and control issues would become a defining part of my personality.

For the next few years, I kept my mother on a very tight leash at Christmas. I continued to enjoy decorating my house inside and out and baking scads of scrumptious cookies, but the whole present thing, even with only ten to open . . . the pit of my stomach would turn.

A few years after that, Dave was in the picture. Our first Christmas together was a little more than a month after our engagement to be married. Now *that* was what Christmas is all about. I brought Dave to a Christmas tree farm where we started our own tradition of picking out the perfect tree. Naturally, each year Dave had to work on his patience because my perfectionism usually made this a fairly lengthy endeavor. He was always amazed by and appreciative of the effort I put into decorating the house both inside and out, and his eyes would glaze over when he saw how many Christmas cookies I baked.

With the decorations in place and the cookies all baked, we'd be ready for the big day. Dave and I always exchanged about a half dozen presents with each other as well as stocking gifts. Eventually, the stress of opening presents started to fade. It took years, but gifts from Dave and gifts from my mother started to evoke entirely different feelings.

I cooked a large, festive meal on just about every Christmas that Dave and I were married. Usually his kids came over, and eventually their spouses and our grandkids came too. A much more meaningful Christmas started to develop: lots of people, cooking, and chatter, plenty of chaos in my perfectly organized world, a variety of Christmas music, abundant memories, and lots and lots and lots of love—piles of love!

Years ago, I started a tradition for Dave and me to watch *It's a Wonderful Life* during the weeks preceding Christmas. I love the story of a desperate man at the end of his rope who decides life is so hopeless that he must take his own life. Yet when there's an opportunity to save someone else, he puts his own misery aside. It's because of the prayers of those who love him that an angel arrives to show him how important his life has been, how his piece of the world and those in it would have been changed forever if he'd never existed. Dave and I watched that movie every year. By the time we'd hear little Zuzu say, "Look, Daddy. Teacher says, every time a bell rings, an angel gets his wings,"[5] I'd be sniffling and sobbing. Dave always chuckled at how emotional I could get over a movie, especially one I'd seen a dozen times! I haven't watched the movie this year. Of all the years, this is the one I really need to watch it. But in the movie, George Bailey develops a new appreciation for the love of his wife, his family, and his community. I feel like that emphasis on the love between spouses is going to bring a whole lot more tears this year.

The last couple of months when Dave was alive, I'd look at the clock and think how fast time was going by. It was like watching sand pour through an hourglass: Its speed never changes, but when there's a lot of sand on the top of the hourglass it looks like the sand is moving slower, and when there are only a few crystals of sand left to fall, it seems it moves so much faster. When I finally accepted our time together was finite, the hours went by so quickly, which is why I spent all my time at home. I think I finally got Dave to understand that.

Now, time ticks by slowly . . . and loudly. My great-great-grandmother's clock that sits in the dining area gets wound every week. It chimes on the hour and the half hour. But the tick-tock of every minute has become frighteningly loud.

When Dave would take his afternoon nap and the house was quiet, I'd try to imagine what it would be like after he was gone. I never really thought about it before then. I could not believe there would come a time when life would be that silent, when Dave wouldn't be taking a nap in the other room. They call it "anticipatory grief." Supposedly, when you experience anticipatory grief, you're preparing yourself for a loss. I came across this sentence in an article I read: "Anticipatory grief is the grief that you expect to experience, much of which is conceptual and can change over time."[6] The key term here is "conceptual." When someone has been loving their person for twenty-two years, they can imagine how they will feel when that person is gone, but they have only a particular frame of reference to use. My dad's death was by far the most significant loss in my life before Dave's death, but in no way does the frame of reference of a ten-year-old girl losing her dad help prepare her for the loss of her husband. *Imagining* Dave was no longer part of my physical life while he napped in the bedroom and I sat in the living room was absolutely nothing like the actual feelings that occurred after he was gone.

Let me try to create a picture of anticipatory grief versus actual grief: Imagine you're afraid of water. Knowing you're going to a pool party in a few weeks, you attempt to conquer this fear by dipping your toe in some water. After a week of this, you go outside in the rain and stand in a puddle. It's awful and you're shaking, but you're surviving it. That's anticipatory grief. Now imagine someone you thought was your friend saying he has a great way for you to get over your fear of water. You happily join him as you both climb into a helicopter, then fly out over the ocean. You're scared because there's no land as far as the eye can see, only water. Then your "friend" pushes you out the door with no life raft or life jacket. He waves as the pilot flies away and leaves you stranded, alone. That's actual grief.

*   *   *

I spent this morning journaling for a few hours while Sadie slept peacefully at the foot of the bed. She's eight years old now and appreciates many good naps throughout the day.

By the time I got moving, nearly half the day was gone. Sadie and I went for a walk, then to the coffee shop. As I walked into the room with the tables, I decided today was going to be the day I sat at our table. Why I picked Christmas Eve to do this is beyond me!

Our table was vacant. As Sadie and I approached it, I told her, "Sadie, we're going to try this . . . not sure how long we'll last."

I sat in the seat I always used to sit in, then positioned Sadie in her usual spot while I stared at Dave's empty seat. I saw him clear as day sitting in that chair and wearing a blue sweatshirt with "Topsail Island" on it. I was shocked I didn't burst into tears. I placed my hand on the table in front of his seat and said out loud, "This isn't as easy as you suggested it would be, you know." Fortunately, it was a quiet day in the coffee shop so there was no one to hear me talking to myself.

Much like anticipatory grief, I don't think Dave had any idea how grieving your person feels. How could he? Lucky for him, he never lost anyone to death. At times I've said, "Dave would have handled this so much better than me," but I think the truth is that Dave would have only *appeared* to handle this better than me because he wouldn't have cried in front of others nor talked about his sadness like I do. But I truly believe at least part of that was because he had no idea how intensely painful this grieving process is every minute of the day. You can't know unless you've done it.

As I stared at his empty seat, I let my mind flash through every memory I have of us in the coffee shop: all the family we brought there . . . all the conversations we had with Jeremy and Tracey . . . all the chats with the gals that work there . . . all the times I reprioritized my day to have coffee with my husband. I just kind of zoned out. It didn't exactly bring me comfort like Dave thought it would, but it didn't make me want to drive off a bridge either . . . so there's that.

When Sadie and I left, we headed to the pet store so I could give her a bath and a blow dry and then indulge in some retail therapy. When we got home, I realized Cathy had reached out to me to ask if I wanted to go for a walk. I missed the walk, but she said she'd come by later. I had managed to stay occupied until a little after 2 p.m. Seven hours down, seven to go. Rinse and repeat.

When Cathy came by, I immersed her in stories and photos of Dave. She'd never been to our house before, and I didn't realize she'd never seen a picture of the pre-cancer, with-a-nose, one-hundred-more-pounds version of Dave. As I gave her a tour of the house, I stopped at Dave's dresser to reminisce over all the photos on it. I changed everything around when Dave started spending more time in bed. I wanted him to be able to see his kids, his grandkids, and me.

There's a picture of us on my fortieth birthday. This photo has been framed for many years but lived in a drawer somewhere until the last month of Dave's life. I love this picture and have no idea why it's been hiding in a drawer rather than being displayed prominently. I said to Cathy, "When I look at Dave in this picture, I can see how much he loves me."

She replied, "That's exactly what I was thinking! It's so obvious."

I went on to say, "This would have been about three years after we were married. I knew I loved my husband, but I didn't know yet how much he loved me, how much that love would enable me to love deeper, how that love would change my life." That's what I see when I look at this picture. I looked so happy because it was my birthday and my loving husband had his arms wrapped around me. Had I known what the next eighteen years would hold, I would have been bursting out of my skin.

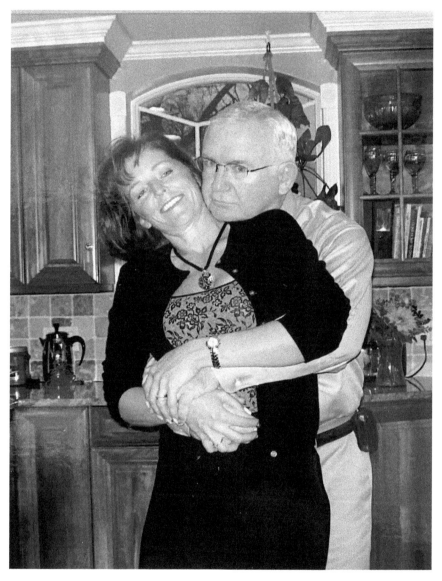

November 2004: My fortieth birthday

*   *   *

Cathy just left and it's nearly 5 p.m., which gives me implied permission for my nightly cocktail. I'm very in tune to the potential for developing a drinking problem. Although I've never relied on alcohol to get me through rough times, with my dad being an alcoholic and that slight numbness that one shot gives me, I can certainly see how a problem could develop. The ever-responsible angel on my shoulder is saying, "You really don't need more problems, Patty, dealing with grief is enough. Only one shot, no more than that." But the rowdy SOB on my other shoulder is saying, "Fuck it. You're a grown-ass woman who lost the love of her life. If you want to drink in the evening to get through the rough times, you do what you gotta do." I'm caught somewhere in the middle of these two extremists sitting on my shoulders.

I'll go ahead and eat dinner and contemplate having a second drink. After all, it's Christmas Eve—

Oh shit! It's Christmas Eve! I forgot what day it is!

A flood of memories of the last twenty-plus years of Christmas Eves with Dave are rushing into my mind. I sense a major meltdown is imminent.

43

Monday, December 25

*T*urns out I had only one drink last night. Then I sat down to watch *It's a Wonderful Life.* I streamed it on some free channel and had to sit through commercials. I could hear Dave in my ear saying, "Why are you sitting through commercials? We have this movie downstairs in my collection." Dave loved to buy DVDs. To me, it was just "more stuff."

The story was beautiful as always. The sentiment that one life affects so many other lives, the lives of people you will never know, is powerful. But when George returns to Bedford Falls after his visit from Clarence, his biggest concern is where his wife is. He longs to see the woman he loves so deeply. Watching that was as painful as I thought it would be.

After watching the movie, I was curious about Jimmy Stewart's life. He was actually a lot like Dave. An incredibly humble man, he enlisted in the US Army Air Force during WWII, participating in several missions and later retiring from the Air Force Reserves as a brigadier general. Stewart met Gloria Hatrick McLean, who was ten years his junior, at a dinner party hosted by Gary Cooper. Stewart said upon meeting her, "I could tell right off that she was a thoroughbred . . . the kind of girl I had always dreamed of. But first I had to woo her dog. I bought him steaks. Patted him. Praised him. It got to be pretty humiliating, but we finally got to be friends. I was free to court Gloria."[7]

I smiled at the similarity of Stewart and McLean's courting process to mine and Dave's. No doubt if Dave had access to my dogs, he would have known wooing them might have shortened the seven-year courting process to something more reasonable. But Dave always said, "Good things are worth waiting for."

After Stewart and McLean married, Stewart adopted McLean's two sons, and they had twin daughters together. McLean had difficulty during the birth, and the hospital staff remembers Stewart to be such a doting and concerned husband. Any of the stories you read about the two of them portray their commitment to one another as apparent to anyone around them, a rarity in the scandalous world of Hollywood. They had been married for forty-four years when McLean succumbed to lung cancer. It's said that after she died, Stewart retreated from public life and secluded himself at home. Reportedly, he opted not to replace the battery in his pacemaker, preferring to let nature take its course. I can only imagine how cheated he felt believing that with his advanced age, he would be the first to go. Three years after McLean's death, Stewart died of a pulmonary embolism. His last words reportedly were, "I'm going to be with Gloria now."[8]

Thinking of Stewart and McLean when I went to bed, I picked up Dave's book to read the last few chapters. I will read his book over and over and over in the years to come. I can hear his voice when I read the words.

Before I turned off the light, I murmured, "If I dream of Dave, please don't make it a painful dream that makes me sad. Please make it one that makes me smile."

Dave and I are on a flight to somewhere. But it doesn't look like the inside of a normal commercial airliner; there's far too much room to move around.

While Dave sits in his seat, I wander off and talk to other passengers. When I come back to him, he asks if I've been off making new friends. He touches his hand to his shoulder while telling me that every time I bend down to talk to someone, my button-down shirt slides off my shoulder, revealing my bra. He's not angry, just a little jealous that someone else is seeing that much skin. I'm surprised he says anything, but I'm secretly flattered he's showing a touch of jealousy.

I bend down to give him a hug. It's a warm, tight hug, the kind that says, "I love you." I know I have only a couple of months left to get these hugs before he goes, so I need to relish them. He mumbles something in my ear, but I don't understand his words. Maybe my ears are clogged from the flight. I lean back, telling him I didn't understand what he said. He responds, "Well, she heard me all the way over there" while pointing to a young lady wearing a white shirt who's sitting about five feet away from us.

At that moment I woke up from the dream. My first words of the day were, "Merry Christmas, Dave. I love you. Thank you for the visit." I still felt satisfied from the warm hug in the dream.

Since finding out Molly is working over the holiday, I've been reaching out to her. This morning I sent her a message saying, "Thinking of you and wondering if any wives will lose their husbands today. I asked God not to take anyone today but realized I was just being selfish. They may want to go." She responded with, "I love you, Patty."

This afternoon I drove to Jeremy and Tracey's for a quiet Christmas. Just some food, a card game, and friends who are like family. Jeremy's house is usually a revolving door of people, and at special gatherings the norm is somewhere between thirty and fifty, often more. But today it was quieter than usual. Only a couple of other friends stopped by to share a Christmas cocktail and a bite to eat.

Later in the day, Bobby popped in. Bobby always smiles when he sees me at Jeremy's house. I remember the day Dave told him "check-out day" was coming soon and asked him to keep an eye on me. Bobby had assured him we were "woven into the fabric of the community." Days like today are what Bobby was talking about. This is what he meant by the community taking care of me.

While sharing laughs and conversation, I had a moment when my mind drifted to the days Dave and I went to Jeremy's together. I'd underestimated the comfort of having the person I love in a social setting. As most couples do, after you say your hellos you drift off to have conversations with small groups of friends. But you always know your person isn't far away, and a knowing glance and a smile from them could mean "Save me from this conversation," "Do you need another drink?" "I'm ready to leave," or "I love you." Thinking of this, my eyes filled with tears.

Jeremy was talking to Bobby when I heard, "Right, Patty?" I was lost in my own thoughts and had no idea what he was talking about. "Umm . . . yeah," I replied, then we made eye contact. He must have been able to see I was having a moment.

When I got home from Jeremy's, I checked in with Molly again via text. I had a slew of questions, and she answered them directly and without violating her patients' and their families' privacy. She was incredibly patient with me. I needed to ask questions about dying people. Somehow it all figures into working out my own grief. I asked her if other wives she's seen are like the way I was with Dave: completely on the bed, very involved with every aspect of his care. I've been curious whether this is how most women support their husband's dying or I'm somewhat unique.

Molly replied, "I have never taken care of a couple who had a love like you and Dave have. I very rarely see someone—you—be so involved and such an advocate and expert in their partner's care. I was surprised to see how wrapped up in bed you were. I loved it. It felt so natural and was beautiful. Holding his hand, your leg over his."

I am so happy she could see that. I am so happy she could *feel* that. I wanted my love for Dave to be the last thing he felt in this world. I am forever changed not only by his life and love for me but by being a part of his death.

Tuesday, December 28

I continue to have flashes of Dave in my head. Sudden, actual glimpses of him. It's like someone puts a flashcard of a memory in front of my eyes. I could be doing anything, thinking of something other than him, when BAM! I see him in my mind. It's startling enough to make me stop whatever I'm doing and continue with the memory. If I'm alone, I often narrate what's going on, almost to affirm it. Many times these incidents turn into crying jags, but if other people are around I often do a quick flick of my head, almost to shake the vision out.

The other night I spoke with Patrick on the phone. I told him I'm researching this whole "God thing" once and for all to determine whether He really could be real. Since Patrick and I are both wired similarly and are both former law enforcement officers, he suggested running it like an investigation makes a lot of sense; build a case and see where the truth lies.

I told him I started reading another book the other day called *The Case for Christ* by Lee Strobel. Prior to writing the book, Mr. Strobel was an award-winning journalist and an atheist. Personal events drove a desire in him to debunk Christianity. Through reliable investigative journalism practices including research and interviews, Strobel aimed to build a case proving that God doesn't exist, the Bible is just a storybook, and the Resurrection of Christ is just malarky. At least, that's what he planned to prove.

Apparently, Strobel and I have a lot in common. But he's done a lot of the work for me, so his story should be helpful in my investigation. Although he's a die-hard nonbeliever, I'm a bit more on the fence.

It turns out the book, which I'm still reading, was made into a movie, and it's terrific! Spoiler alert: As you might suspect, Mr. Strobel is unable to prove his beliefs, and ultimately the evidence sways him to a life as a believer in Christ. And not just a believer, but he ultimately dedicates his life to pastoring.

As I watched the movie, some ideas resonated with me. When Strobel interviews an agnostic psychologist with a lot of street cred, the doctor nonchalantly asks him whether he has a good relationship with his father, which it turns out he doesn't. She informs him that many of the well-known atheists, such as Hume, Nietzsche, Sartre, and Freud, all had a father who either died when they were young, abandoned them, or was physically or emotionally abusive. In the world of therapy, she says, this is called a "father wound." Strobel suggests that just because he doesn't have a father who loves him doesn't mean he can't accept that there is a father who loves all of us.

I paused and gave this a moment of thought, being that my dad was physically and emotionally unavailable to me.

Since much of Strobel's research hinges on whether the Crucifixion and Resurrection happened, he seeks out all types of professionals, including theologists, medical doctors, historians, and even an archaeologist-turned-Catholic priest. When he asks one of them, "Why would Jesus die on the cross?" the simple answer is, "Love."

Hearing this hit me like a ton of bricks. As a child hearing "Jesus died for your sins," I wondered the same thing as Strobel. Why would this gentle man named Jesus not run away? Why would He allow this to happen? I find the answer being love is so simple, yet so powerful. Until Dave, I didn't really understand the power of love. And it wasn't until the last two weeks of his life that I truly learned I would do anything for Dave—absolutely anything—in the name of love.

Strobel continues to seek evidence to prove his atheist beliefs. But the more he searches, the more his research leans towards proving what he wanted to disprove. A coworker asks him, "When is enough evidence enough evidence?"

This made me think back to the morning after Dave's death: Margaret, Patrick, and I stopping to help a sloth-like turtle on our way to the funeral home, "Somewhere Over the Rainbow" playing at the coffee shop, and a loose dog running around the road. These are all things Dave would definitely do if he were, in fact, a spirit trying to get my attention. Margaret had believed these to be signs from Dave, but I'd told her they were just coincidences and relayed my knowledge on "clear and convincing evidence" in the eyes of the law. But *when is enough evidence enough evidence?*

By the time the movie was over, I was puzzled and a little bit speechless. Why didn't I start this "God journey" with Dave while he was still here? This is a rhetorical question, as I know the answer: It is *because* of Dave's death that I am seeking these answers.

My newfound focus wouldn't surprise Dave at all. He knew and would often say I could be like a dog with a bone when I became focused. Whether it's tenacity, grit, or OCD, once I start something, I don't stop until I finish.

Could God actually be real? If so, this is huge!

While doing some further research, I came upon C. S. Lewis again. The name is familiar to me because he's the author of that quote I found after Bobby and I walked and talked for two hours. I pulled up the quote, the one about God rebuilding your decent little cottage into a palace so He can dwell in it Himself. How surprising to read that C. S. Lewis became an atheist at the age of fifteen and had a distant, demanding, and eccentric father. Yet later in life, he's quoted as saying, "Christianity is a statement which, if false, is of no importance, and if true, of infinite importance. The one thing it cannot be is moderately important."[9]

This is exactly what I've been saying! If you spend your life as a believer, benefiting from the comfort of the thought that a Heavenly Father exists, there is no downside. If you die and you're wrong, you will never know. No harm, no foul.

But what if it's true?

My head is spinning in all different directions. I will continue to seek out my truth.

44

Sunday, December 31

So tomorrow is the first day of the new year. Most people who aren't in the middle of a crisis at the turn of the year are busy listing their annual resolutions: losing weight, quitting smoking, being more mindful . . . the usual crap. Mine will be the same tomorrow as it was yesterday: continue to try to put one foot in front of the other.

I knew mornings would be difficult. When Dave was still here, I thought about how I would dread the mornings after he died. Now that I have exactly sixty-three mornings under my belt, I can say with some certainty that mornings are no worse than any other time of the day.

Seeing half the bed empty is a pretty lonesome way to start the day, but the biggest problem with mornings is waking with a sense of dread and feeling like I'm starring in the movie *Groundhog Day*. Every morning is encumbered with the feeling of, "How do I get through another day?" It's like I'm just biding my time. And the vulnerability in the morning is awful. I get smacked in the head a half dozen times a day with the cruel reminder that Dave is gone, but somehow when it happens before I've even fluttered my eyes open, had my first sip of coffee, or even taken my morning pee, it seems unusually harsh. Couple that with it occurring on the heels of a dream, and just starting the day can present multiple hurdles.

That being said, maybe mornings *are* worse than other times of the day. I don't know. It all sucks.

The other morning, I woke up with a pain in my breast. It was the oddest thing really, as I've never felt a throb there before. This clearly wasn't a sore boob from sleeping wrong. I reached into my tank top to see whether it felt different. Nothing unusual. For a moment I lay there with my mind racing. Then I said out loud while staring up at the ceiling, "You've got to be fucking kidding me. If I get breast cancer I'll be so pissed off." I know jumping from a throbbing boob to breast cancer is a significant stretch, but it did cross my mind.

The other thing that crossed my mind is that I don't know whether I would treat it. I know that breast cancer is one of the more "curable" cancers to treat, but I'm not sure I'd want to. Maybe this would be a way out. Then I wondered if I didn't treat it and six months later it metastasized, would there be a time I'd look back and be really annoyed at myself for not taking control when it was first detected? Is it possible that when the sands of the hourglass we call life draw down to the final grains, I would have a sudden desire to stick around? If there's any chance in the world that Dave can see me and he saw that I didn't treat breast cancer, he would be really upset. After the way I advocated for him, he would be incredibly sad to see I didn't do the same for myself.

And that's another thing. I'm sick of constantly worrying about disappointing Dave. I hardly ever worried about disappointing him during the last twenty-two years we were together, but ever since he died I think about it all the time. I know Dave and I talked about WWDD, but that was meant not so much for action-type decisions but more so for dealing with people. I tend to be a bit . . . eh . . . let's just say that sugarcoating is not my strong suit. Dave didn't BS people, but he had a gentleness that doesn't exactly come natural to me—unless I'm thinking WWDD.

*　　*　　*

We had about five inches of nonstop rain the other day. When it finally stopped and I took Sadie outside for a walk, I thought I should probably take a peek in the camper. I had no reason to think there was water inside, but it never hurts to look.

I can't emphasize enough how much I love our little camper. I used to ask Dave all the time on our trips, "Isn't this the cutest camper? Don't you just love it?" He'd laugh and appease my questions by agreeing with me and saying he loves the "tin can." With all its coziness, it was homey and comfy on those wet, foggy, or cold days. I always thought the cozy factor came from all the modifications and decorations—curtains, comfy bedding, happy dog, steaming cup of coffee—wrong. The cozy factor came from the love inside.

I don't know how I will ever be able to take the camper out again. Even if I can take it to the nearby mountains for a few days of hiking, I seriously can't see how I'll travel the country in it. Dave would be mortified! On his deathbed he was concerned about coming up with camping companions for me. He knew this would be a way for me to create happiness in my life.

When I walked into the camper, I saw the canvas prints on the wall from our BLTs and thought of the shakes I made for Dave with limited counter space, the naps he took under his air force blanket, the movies we watched, the times we hung out at the dinette while each of us worked on our respective blogs, and all the snuggles we enjoyed. The camper has two twin beds, and at times not only did we snuggle in one of them but Sadie joined us as well. It was pretty humorous because no one could move once we were all in place.

I thought of all the trips I planned with Dave in mind, which meant nothing too strenuous, but there were sights to see, downtowns to visit, coffee shops to stop at, and historical sites to explore. I planned anything related to air and space for Dave and places like the Johnny Carson Gallery or the largest working weathervane for me. I must admit, I pretty much planned and executed each trip with Dave's quality of life 100 percent in the forefront of my mind. I wanted him happy and as comfortable as he could be but not entirely exhausted. When I accomplished *that*, I considered it to be a successful trip.

But now, what good is planning sightseeing events? Who am I going to share them with? When I planned the BLTs, I said to Dave, "I want you with me when I see these things for the first time." Well, I want him with me when I see all things for the first time. And Dave was no different. When he was healthy and went to a new town or city by himself, he always came home telling me how he saw this place or that restaurant and wanted to take me there. That's what makes something special . . . sharing it with someone you love.

*   *   *

I'm not officially listening to music again, but I have taken a liking to NPR radio, which I find rather ironic since I've never listened to it in my life. I suppose this is part of creating a new normal. It seems to keep my mind occupied and doesn't evoke the same emotions most music seems to bring on. Although, I was mindlessly scrolling through social media the other day when a tune caught my ear. It was classical music, something Dave nor I ever listened to, unless you count *Phantom of the Opera*. It may have been the most beautiful song I've ever heard.

I glanced at the artist and pulled up the song in its entirety on a music streaming service: "Passacaglia" by Roman Nagel, a composer and pianist. The melody takes my breath away! Dave would love it. I'm so sad I can't share it with him. I searched through all the other songs by this artist and selected two others that spoke to me: "Blue Waltz" and "Unconditional Love."

Once a day, I choose to sit and listen to these three songs and cry, accompanied by memories of Dave. How I wish I could share this music with him.

My big New Year's Eve activity will be my nightly cocktail, then dinner, a hot bath, and the usual television. I expect to have the lights out by 10 p.m., pretty much the same as my recent New Year's Eves with Dave.

I tend to take more baths in the colder months. Naturally they always make me think of Dave now. Our routine Tub Talks towards the end of his life were a very intimate part of each day. I've still been sitting on the end of the tub with the fixture. I knew this would happen. I knew I would never want to revert to sitting in the tub "the normal way" after tubbing with Dave. Lately I've been sitting in the short direction. That's got to be the stupidest thing I've heard. Instead of sitting north/south, I've been sitting east/west with my legs folded. Just dumb. Dave would tell me, "Cut the shit and sit in the tub so you're comfortable." Those would be his exact words. Tonight I slipped into the tub "the right way." I thought back to the days I used to tub sitting in this direction. That was before.

I glanced at the wall in front of me and saw the shelf that I haven't really looked at since the last time I sat in this direction, which was at least six months ago. On the shelf sits a vase we were given by a friend of Dave's for our wedding, a wooden frog lounging on his side from one of our vacations, an unused candle decorated with shells, and little glass figurines given to me by my dear friend Lisa who passed away at the age of forty. Then there's the sign I made at that girl's night painting party soon after Dave and I moved here, when we were having difficulties. The host had supplied all the tools and the guests selected their canvases and paints. I chose a wood board, some shells, and a bunch of paint, then scrolled online looking for inspiration. Once I found the perfect quote, I replicated it: "You can't stop the waves, but you can learn to surf." Seemed appropriate for the time of life I was in when I found it. I think I could apply that to my life now, although I still feel like I've been hit by something resembling a tsunami more than just a wave.

Sitting in this direction lasted less than a minute before I spun around 180 degrees. That was better. That's what I'm familiar with now.

Tonight, on the last night of the year, my mind recollected everything that happened in this room in 2023—the good, the bad, and the ugly. My phone was in reach, and I pulled up the songs by Nagel; they total just under nine minutes. I sank down into the tub and let my mind wander. The tears flowed freely. I will now call this music, "Nine Minutes of Tears."

45

Thursday, January 4

On New Year's Day, I had some ambition to do closet reorganizing, which is generally my go-to coping mechanism. Whenever I'd clean closets and drawers, Dave would ask why it was that only his stuff got tossed. "Well, I don't keep half the crap you keep," I'd tease. In truth, I never threw out anything of his. But I do like things streamlined and tidy. Closets that allow me to reach in and grab what I want without having to rummage around are very satisfying to me. I'm sure there are some control issues loosely tied in there.

I've still barely touched anything of Dave's since he died. While in the closet looking at his clothes, books, coins, and other items he cared enough about to keep in our bedroom closet, I thought of our discussions concerning "stuff." We both agreed stuff is just stuff. If it can be bought with money, it's not valuable. It may be expensive, but not valuable. Valuables are your kids' projects from thirty years ago and greeting cards given to each other over the last twenty-two years.

Sometime during the last five years, when I felt the cost of greeting cards becoming prohibitive, I started rummaging through Dave's "keep-it box" when a card-giving occasion came up. For each upcoming occasion, I'd pick out the perfect card that I'd given him in the past, cross out the previous date, and replace it with the current year. Then I'd make a fancy envelope for the card. Dave got such a kick out of it. The last time I did that was this past August 18 . . . his birthday. He laughed and laughed and shook his head at how much effort I'd made to save the $7.99 that I would have spent on a new greeting card. I told him, "Why spend all that money when I bought you such a perfect card three years ago?" You can't fight that kind of logic.

I'm still not ready to start tossing the stuff that has no emotional attachment, though I am ready to give things to the people Dave would want them to go to or to people who could use them. But as long as some of his stuff gives me comfort, it can stay right where it is. And I'll keep wearing his pajama bottoms.

*   *   *

After my little burst of energy on the first of the year, I kind of hit a road bump. It feels like someone put a wet blanket over me. I just feel . . . heavy. It's not like I'm crying all the time, as I'm still functioning and appear to the world that I'm coping well, but I just feel weighted, and I'm wondering how long it will last.

I'm still having my nightly shot of bourbon. I made the mistake the other night of having more than one. I'm not really sure how much I drank, but it was enough that I realized it wasn't a good idea. By the last sip of the first shot, the painful edges of grief are slightly sanded down to rounded corners. Bumping into the grief still bruises, but it doesn't cut through the skin. However, several shots of spirits? Ugh. That just made me cry. Full-on sloppy crying.

As I made my morning coffee today, I looked at the whiteboard on my fridge. For years this whiteboard has reminded me of information such as my meal planning for the week, and over the last six months it's where I wrote the ever-changing pain management schedule for Dave. These days, it has a bit of advice from me to me, which I came up with one day when getting to the next hour seemed impossible:

ONE

One breath

One moment

One day

One foot in front of the other

After wondering what to do with the rest of my day, I decided to sit at the kitchen counter and do a bit of research. I'm still in the middle of reading two books revolving around confirmation that God exists and that NDEs are proof that the death of the physical body is not the end of the soul. But I've started wondering, with all this interpretation of data, why hasn't anyone said what percentage of clinical deaths per year result in resuscitation? And out of those resuscitations, how many result in NDEs? Because if only .001 percent of clinical deaths result in an NDE, I'm not going to find that very clear and convincing.

I was having no luck looking for the numbers I was searching for. I'm not a professional at this, but I am known for my dogged determination. So I figured maybe I should start looking at the other side's argument; maybe I should start reading what the naysayers have to say if I want to make an educated decision about God and the hereafter. I came upon just such an article, and I didn't have to look for long. It basically confirms what my thoughts and fears have been. One explanation for an NDE is that it occurs when the brain releases a ketamine-like substance that affects a person's perception of being separate from their body, which leads to hallucinations.[10] If the person is resuscitated after this experience, they might have a memory of an NDE. But what if the person is unable to be resuscitated? If this experience is all produced by the brain, then I imagine if the body is not resuscitated, the lights go out. Permanently.

I don't know what to think. It's only one article, but it suggests that my skepticism is directed exactly where it should be. Believing would be so comforting, but how do you make yourself believe something your gut is telling you is wrong?

Although there may not be any clear and convincing evidence as to what happens to us after we die, the one message I keep coming across in these books is that our purpose while we are here is to *love* one another. I know this doesn't just mean loving Dave. So when I saw my mother the other day, a visit I initiated, I told her that I'm willing to try to have a relationship with her while still maintaining my boundaries but that it's extremely important to me she makes an effort to filter her words. So far it seems to be working. We're doing well together. Better than usual.

I asked my mother the same question I've been asking myself: "If you knew you had only one year to live, would you live your life differently?"

I think I gave her something to consider.

✳   ✳   ✳

I went to Jaiden's graduation party this afternoon, but I needed something to do until then. I called Nancy from the nail salon to see if she could squeeze me in. She could, but I needed to wait awhile, so I grabbed the book I'm reading and sat in front of the Food Lion, reading about God and the afterlife while I waited. I think Dave would be amused to see all the changes in me that he created; carrying a book in the car is so unlike me. I'm sure he would also be saddened, although probably not surprised, by my sadness and difficulty in accepting his death.

Ten minutes before my appointment, I put down the book and went inside the nail salon. Nancy was on the phone and motioned for me to sit down at her station. They often play a Bossa Nova radio station on YouTube. It's basically every song you've ever heard, everything from ballads to rock, played in a Muzak-y type of manner, but the songs have lyrics and that's the only way you'd recognize them. I found it rather amusing hearing a Guns N' Roses song in this style.

While Nancy continued her conversation at the back of the room, I suddenly noticed the song that was playing: "I Can't Help Falling in Love." Geez. The song I was supposed to have at my wedding, the one I forgot I wanted to have as our wedding song, the one I remembered after Dave and I got married. We had several laughs about that. With no one nearby, I said out loud, "That's just a coincidence. That song being played means nothing."

Nancy finished her call and sat down opposite me. She asked how I was doing, and I told her what I tell everyone: "I'm taking one day at a time." As she started working on my nails, I listened to the music. The song playing was "Somewhere Over the Rainbow." My mind raced. *Is this just a coincidence? It's just two songs. Two significant songs, but just two songs.* My mind continued to steamroll along, convincing me that two songs didn't prove anything.

Five minutes or so passed, and I heard the next song: "From This Moment On." Our wedding song. The song playing when Dave shouldered my weight after I froze up during the first dance.

Three songs. Three very significant songs. What are the odds this playlist would have these three songs *and* be playing when I decided to have an impromptu manicure? The odds were small enough that my eyes filled with tears and a smile came across my face.

Nancy was busily working on my nails and was unaware of the revelation I was having: Could this really be happening?

Could Dave actually *be*? Is God real? Are prayers heard? Is this really a sign created by Dave? It would be so like him to throw me two significant songs and then a third when I'm struggling to believe the first two.

I was still smiling after I left. I feel this event will affect the rest of my life. Isn't that the strangest thing?

As I drove to Jaiden's party, I felt a little spring in my step, a little pep. The wet blanket has been peeled off me just a bit.

When I got to the party, Jaiden came running out looking adorable at the young age of seventeen. She gave me a huge hug and told me she was sitting with the "DG girls," the girls from the coffee shop. Each of them got up and gave me a warm hug when I got to the table . . . just like they would have if Dave were there.

I enjoyed the next hour or so hanging out with the girls who could all be my daughters, some even my granddaughters. On the tables were heart-shaped cards on which guests could write their words of wisdom for the graduate. Being that I've spent some time thinking lately, I asked myself, *If I'd known then what I know now, what would I tell my seventeen-year-old self?* Dave and I discussed this only months ago, and I knew exactly what to write:

> You are enough. Pretty enough, smart enough, strong enough.

> Continue to be kind. Your kindness goes a long way in making a difference in people's lives.

> Love is what makes the world go 'round. Love hard.

I told Jaiden to save this card and pull it out in thirty years. She'll be forty-seven and I'll be gone. "Think back to this day, and I bet you'll see that it was good advice," I told her. I can't even imagine how much living she has in front of her.

When I left the gathering of girls, I was still smiling. I told Dave if I can really believe he "is," then I'm going to start sharing everything with him. I'm going to talk to him all the time. Isn't that wonderful?

"Don't throw me in that briar patch," he would say.

46

Friday, January 5

*C*hris-from-the-beach sent me a reel that she made for social media today to wish her husband a happy birthday in Heaven. She's hoping Jim sends her a big sign today. I spent the day wondering whether Chris ever received her sign from Jim.

This evening I received an inquiry from a woman regarding a grill I listed for sale on Facebook Marketplace. I'd just picked up my phone and was heading to bed when the message came through. I told her it was still available, and as I waited for her reply, I clicked on her profile to see who I was dealing with. Ironically, Snoop Dog is incredibly vague on social media; I don't even use my real name, and I have my privacy settings high. I'm often surprised by those who let the world see everything about themselves. I saw the woman had a couple of reviews posted, and one was for a psychic medium. Hmm. I put all this "medium nonsense" out of my head after watching the one on Zoom who was trying to beef up her business with free readings; I was really disgusted when I read about her budding scammer reputation. But as with any profession, there will always be scammers and those who fall prey to scams.

I asked my potential buyer about the medium, and she said she'd been very impressed with him. I figure I'll ask her more questions tomorrow when I meet her for the grill exchange.

Saturday, January 6

Today I went about my day still riding on the coattails of the excitement I felt when I heard those three significant songs during my manicure. It opens the possibility that Dave still IS. If Dave IS, then God IS, and that's huge. Naturally, the void in my days is still immense, but this does put a different spin on things. In the end game, it would mean that I will see Dave again. Believing in that would make coping a possibility.

While preparing to meet the lady who's buying my grill, I pulled up the psychic's website and watched a video of his story. It included basic info such as when he became a medium, what exactly he does, and what to expect during a reading. He does virtual readings and the price is reasonable. If I do this, it's going to be a "one and done" for me. Whether it's a good reading or a bad reading, I am not going to spend my life lining the pockets of psychics with my dollars.

When I met the woman to sell the grill, I asked her a few quick questions about the medium. She said she really liked the guy. After I returned home, I started cooking dinner while still tossing around the idea of scheduling a reading. What the heck. Yes! I decided I'm going to do it.

I sat down at my Mac and noticed the big apple on the screen. What? I wondered why that would be, as it only reboots during an update. I waited for the reboot to complete and got a message that certain programs could not open because the date and time were wrong. *How could that be? My Mac is set to automatically know the date and time.* As I went into the settings to figure out the problem, I noticed the time was about an hour and a half off and the date was set to October 6, 2021. Weird. I shut it down, counted to ten, and rebooted. Again, the date appeared as October 6, 2021.

After some troubleshooting with Apple, I finally got the computer back to normal. But I started wondering whether this was a sign that I shouldn't make an appointment with the medium. These days, I'm trying to be more open-minded to following the path I'm supposed to travel. Whether it's God, Dave, the universe, or some combination of them all, I'm trying to consider that coincidence may not be just coincidence. The fact that someone showed interest in my grill, and in the winter, and that that person reviewed a psychic medium . . . isn't there a possibility I'm supposed to follow that path? But maybe the computer whacked out because I'm not. I didn't know what to think.

I reached out to Chris, figuring she's the one friend crazy enough to help me make some sense of whether to schedule a session with this psychic and interpret whether my Mac malfunction, something that had never happened before, was a sign. We FaceTimed, and she sat quietly while I told her the entire story.

"So, the date was October sixth?" she confirmed.

"Yes," I replied, "it was the weirdest thing. I even pulled up my calendar. Nothing of significance happened on October sixth, 2021, or any other October sixth," I replied.

Chris looked contemplative and said, "Patty, October sixth was my wedding anniversary. I wonder if Jim was sending me a sign through you."

This is all so baffling! Of all the dates that could have popped up on my computer, there's less than a dozen that would have been of significance to Chris or to me. Yet out of 365 possible dates, one of them did pop up. On top of that, although the date wasn't significant to me, it was significant to the one person I reached out to.

Chris was smiling because she felt she got her sign. She'd been feeling a little disappointed since nothing came yesterday. Once again, I'm more convinced Chris and I meeting on the beach that night was not random. I'm also realizing how much our lives are affected by one another.

When we got off the phone, I scheduled a virtual session with the psychic medium for the first date he has available: March 2.

Wednesday, January 10

I'm still on my quest regarding God and the afterlife. I've read about a half dozen books now, more than I've read in the last ten years. I'm so "religion ignorant." I used to repeatedly ask Dave questions like, "What's an epistle?" "What's the difference between the New Testament and the Old Testament?" "What does 'evangelical' mean?" These are just some of the basics of theism I could never remember. Although Dave was once an altar boy in a Catholic mass performed in Latin, as he got older he was not a believer of religion. He thought religion had become too much about money and power and not enough about God. He used to say, "Look how many wars have been started in the name of religion."

I know Dave and Pastor Bobby spoke about God's existence. I wish Dave and I had spoken more about it. Why didn't we? I couldn't have anticipated that I would have this need to know about God like I do now, but I do think Dave believed in God. Actually, I'm pretty certain he believed. He just wasn't 100 percent certain, and he was okay with that. I envy that Dave didn't have the need for certainty and was content with his belief.

We're all different when it comes to believing in things without proof, but I think all people would fit into three categories in this regard. If you asked one hundred people the question "What would you do if you were told not to touch a park bench because it was just painted and the paint is still wet?" ninety-eight of them would respond in one of two ways: (1) saying, "Geez. Thanks. I won't touch it," and (2) saying, "Really? The paint is wet?" while sticking out an index finger, being satisfied only when their fingertip is covered in paint.

Then there's the type like me, one of only two people whose response to a warning of wet paint would be, "Really? When did you paint? What kind of paint is it, latex or oil-based? When do you expect it to be dry? Is it the first coat or the second coat?" I know . . . annoying. I even annoy myself. But I love logical, concrete proof. It puts me at ease. The scientist in me would say, "I'm wired that way." The person of faith would say, "God made you that way." I wonder whether both can be right.

In the most recent book I read, *A Grief Observed* by C. S. Lewis, I found so many points I could identify with that I wondered how Lewis was able to get inside my head and publish this book three years before I was born. One of the most impactful was this: "I once read the sentence 'I lay awake all night with toothache, thinking about toothache and about lying awake.' That's true to life. Part of every misery is, so to speak, the misery's shadow or reflection: the fact that you don't merely suffer but have to keep on thinking about the fact that you suffer. I not only live each endless day in grief, but live each day thinking about living each day in grief."[11]

Truer words were never said.

Tonight I went to a town meeting and spoke during the part of the meeting that's open to the public, something I used to do quite often when Dave and I attended them monthly. This is the first one I've spoken at since Dave died. It felt lonely not having him sitting in the chair next to me. How could I be in a roomful of people yet still feel that void? When Dave was there, if nothing else I knew I had one fan in the room, my teammate on a two-person team.

I wanted to make a suggestion to the town that they offer a drop-off location for battery recycling. I know fairly well most of the eight people who sit on the dais, so when it was my turn to speak, I thought a joke was in order. I said with a smirk, "The buzzwords that will often gain my attention are "animals" and "environment," for which my late husband probably would have called me a right-wing tree hugger." Most of these eight people knew Dave, so there were a few chuckles. I continued speaking for the three minutes the public is allotted.

As I drove home in the dark by myself, I thought how Dave would have gotten a chuckle out of that comment. I wish I could have heard his laughter.

Thursday, January 11

This morning I woke up in the darkness about an hour earlier than I have for the last ten weeks. My first thought was of a convoluted dream I'd just had. But there was one part of that dream that made me smile:

> I'm driving home from the town meeting and looking forward to telling Dave about my clever comment. When I see him, I say, "So this is what I said to the council: 'My late husband—that's when I thought you were dead—probably would have called me a right-wing tree hugger.'"

In the dream, it didn't seem weird saying to Dave, "When I thought you were dead." I never got to hear Dave's response, but it was a complete relief to dream of Dave and not start the day with overwhelming sadness. Instead of my usual first words of the day being, "Good morning, Dave, I love you," today's words were, "That was pretty funny, don't you think?" as a small giggle slipped out.

I got out of bed knowing I had an extra hour to fill today, and I was actually okay with it. Most of the day passed with thoughts of Dave being frequent but brief, much the way a moth touches a lightbulb. By evening, I wanted some "Dave time." I lay on the living room floor with Sadie and played

"Nine Minutes of Tears," which has become my go-to for when I want to think about Dave, feel the sadness, and have the space to cry. Tears, another name for unused love, leaked out the way they always do.

I followed the nine minutes with a quick tub. Sitting in the end I've been sitting in for the last few months, I looked up at the ceiling and said, "No, I'm not going to sit at the normal end of the tub. Not today, not tomorrow, and probably—"

That's about as far as I got when I realized those words sounded so familiar to me. It's almost the same as the mantra that kept me sane when I feared losing Dave: "He's here today, he'll probably be here tomorrow, and more than likely the day after that."

I've said those words so often over three years, how could this be the first time I've even thought of them in the last ten weeks?

47

Monday, January 15

I visited my mother on Saturday. I actually spent about three hours with her, just talking. That should be proof enough that Dave is a spirit watching over me. In the last thirty years, it has been virtually impossible to talk to my mother for that long without any tension, at least not unless Dave was present to serve as a buffer.

I shared with her every single sign I have received that could have been from Dave. That in itself is a huge deal. I've often regretted sharing personal matters with my mother. Let's hope this time is different.

I told her about the books and the television series I've been watching about God. My mother was raised Lutheran, but she hasn't gone to church with any regularity in at least forty years. About ten years ago, some online "friends" swayed her away from believing in God. I'm not quite sure why a rational person would want to make someone not believe. I've always thought it to be such a personal decision.

And I shared with her the one common theme in my "God research" that keeps coming up over and over. Surprisingly, I told her, it's not the commandments, the disciples, or the Bible stories. Nor is it sin, Heaven and Hell, or judgment day. It's love. Maybe the fact that this one recurring theme keeps coming up means that love really does make the world go 'round.

But this morning was rough. Just as I was focused on Dave's nutrition, I'm now focused on mine. I eat pretty healthy most of the time, but somehow I screwed up my meals yesterday and basically ended up eating a box of raisin bran for dinner while sitting in front of the TV. And I mean, nearly an entire box of raisin bran. Reminiscent of the days of disordered eating, I mindlessly moved my hand from box to mouth, dumping flakes and raisins into my mouth for hours. I knew I'd pay for this. I barely slept at all.

Between my stomach being unhappy and general insomnia, it was an awful night. I woke up on Dave's side of the bed at my normal time after having finally managed a couple of hours of solid sleep. My stomach was still tormented by all the bran. My intestines were speaking to me. I looked in the direction you would look if someone were standing bedside. I remembered the morning I came in to wake Dave when I could smell something wasn't right.

As I lay on his side of the bed, looking at my imaginary face looking down at him, I wondered what he was feeling when I told him what had happened. What an awful moment for Dave! What was he thinking? Did he just want it all to be over? Was he embarrassed? Was he regretting putting me through this when all I could think of was what he was going through? So, this morning when I said, "Good morning, Dave, I love you," I also said, "I'm so sorry you had to go through that. I'm so sorry it was so awful for you. I really had no idea what was happening nor what to expect."

Yesterday I started toying with the idea of taking some RV trips this year. I don't actually want to travel anywhere now. Traveling is another one of those things that I totally misjudged when I thought I knew how I'd react to Dave's death. I was sure

I'd want to pack up the camper and head out for six months to be alone. Okay, maybe that's an exaggeration, but it was the general idea. This couldn't have been further from the truth.

I'm now cringing over the idea of not being able to share new places with Dave. I struggle so much every day not having him here for the mundane details of my life; without him, how will I cope with more significant events such as visiting the World's Largest Ice Cream Cone? And I knew this would be a problem. This was one thing I got absolutely right about anticipating the worst parts of Dave dying.

In March, I plan to spend a week in the mountains of Georgia with Teddy. Of Megan's three boys, he's definitely the one who'll enjoy this the most. I imagine I may have to upgrade my earplugs because the boy will talk your ears off, but I expect it'll be fun. Still, I need to plan a very short, rip-the-bandage-off trip before that. I need time to cry and grieve while being in the camper without Dave. And I need to do that alone. I'm hoping we have some mild weather in February, so maybe I'll take the camper and Sadie a couple of hours away from home and just wallow in it.

I've also started poking around online looking for a place to go in August. It's so damned humid here. Dave and I started making August a mandatory travel month, so I may as well keep up the tradition. I'm thinking this trip needs to be something that Dave would never have wanted to do. I'm sure I will still miss him not being able to share in my enjoyment, but it might make it easier if it's something *he* wouldn't enjoy.

I keep thinking back to a conversation we had a year or two ago. We'd just left the hospital and were headed home on our three-hour drive via backroads. At this point, I hadn't really considered Dave dying. I knew intellectually it was going to happen someday, and I'd read everything there was to read about this vulgar, insidious disease. But I hadn't given a single thought to what life would look like without my husband.

Dave asks me, "So, what are you going to do after I croak?"

That's my Dave.

"Well," I respond, "I suppose the one thing I won't do is make any major decisions. I won't plan on moving or listing the house for at least a year."

He supports my rational thinking by replying, "That makes sense."

I figure he must want more. I would. I would want more if I asked that question. "I imagine I will plan some road trips with the camper that are more tailored to my likes," I add.

He seems happy with that response.

What I didn't realize at the time I answered that question is that I was looking only at the big picture and thinking about what big plans I could make. I certainly wasn't considering how I'd survive the day-to-day "after Dave croaks." Even if I had, I never could have said to him, "Well, I imagine I will wonder if my life has purpose without you and struggle to get through twenty-four hours that feel like forty-eight."

When we first retired to North Carolina, I was bored to tears. That's when I started rescuing birds as a first responder for a local bird rescue. Initially, there were so many hours in the day to fill that spending two to three hours capturing a bird, driving to the rescue facility, and returning home was a welcome diversion. Sometimes Dave even came with me for the ride. I've barely rescued any birds over the last year. With the bird hospital being nearly forty miles away, I never wanted to be that far from Dave, but I also didn't have a couple of hours to spare.

Well, today I received a notification on my phone about a loon stranded on the beach. I love loons! I need to get back to doing things that make me feel good. I remember receiving that beautiful letter Arleen wrote to me after Dave died that said, "Rescue a bird, rescue a dog, go rescue something. That's what you do." She's such a wonderful lady and has been like a mother to me almost since the day I met her, hence the reason I call her Mum.

As is often the case, the evenings are particularly difficult. Mandy gave me a good visual description of grief: Imagine a room. In that room is a box that represents grief. In the beginning, the box is almost the same size as the room. Because there's no space around the box, you constantly bump into it. But as time goes on, more space grows around the box to maneuver without hitting the grief.

Great. But what about when I do hit the box? When I bump into grief, it feels just like the first time. It hurts. So the hurt will hurt hard whenever I bump into the box, it's just that I'll bump into it less often.

48

Wednesday, January 17

*I*t's funny how two people can look at the same object and see it in two completely different ways. Much like the glass half empty/glass half full analogy, both people are right, it's just that their perspectives are different.

It's much the same with coincidence and what I'll call "God winks." These little serendipities that take place throughout the day need some explaining. I'm quite convinced that a coincidence is a God wink minus faith. When there's no explanation for good things that happen, especially when they don't seem scientifically probable, we define them as coincidences. But what about when the odds are rare? Is it an unlikely coincidence then?

On Sunday, Cathy sent me a text with a link to a church that gives sermons she listens to on YouTube. She sent it to me last week, and I enjoyed the pastor and told her so. There's no pressure in her texts, as she knows I'm trying to find my way at my own pace, but she wants to give me a hand if I'm willing to take it. The pastor is a little like Bobby in that you don't have to be a decades-long churchgoer to follow his sermons. I started listening to the most recent sermon last night before bed and couldn't keep my eyes open for the last half hour.

This morning I had an appointment with Mandy. With my latte in hand, I streamed the second half of the sermon while I drove to see her. One of the topics discussed was prayer, and the pastor used the term "pray" as an acronym. Being that I'm such a visual person and someone who likes instruction (I don't like to "wing it"), this seemed like it might be right up my alley.

The letter P is for praise. I'm probably not as good at praising the Lord as I should be. As I drove, I told Him I'm sorry I'm not tripping over myself with praise for Him because I'm still struggling with His existence.

The letter R is for repent. This is when we say we're sorry for our sins. As I was driving, I thought about what my sins are. The first things that came to mind were things that followed the words "Thou shalt not." I really couldn't think of much. Ultimately, I said I'm sorry that I don't even know what my sins are, even though I'm sure I have some.

The letter A is for ask. This is usually what my entire prayers consist of. I asked for all the things that I usually ask for when I pray: to make Himself more visible to me, to be a greater presence in my life, to make the burden of grief easier, and to please, please take care of Dave and please—whether it's God or whether it's Dave—please send me more signs.

The letter Y is for yield. We must yield to the voice of the Holy Spirit. I drove quietly, listening intently in my head. Listening. Nothing. Listening harder. Nothing still. And then some words just popped into my head: "I'm here. Believe in me." Whether it was wishful thinking or the Holy Spirit, I don't know.

By the time I pulled into Mandy's parking lot, I felt fairly spent from the prayer. I had about ten minutes to sit in her waiting area before my appointment, so I pulled out my phone and started scrolling through Facebook. Within seconds, one of those targeted ads showed up on my stream. I'm not quite sure what algorithm picked this for me . . . or maybe it wasn't Facebook . . . maybe it was a God wink. The ad was for an adorable gift of a cuddly stuffed critter. The critter was in a pretty blue box with the words "Someone Loves You" written on the side of the box and an artificial blue rose tucked inside. Well, I've always loved blue flowers, but what struck me most was the critter . . . it was a plush sloth.

Ten minutes after I prayed for signs to continue, an ad came up on my feed with Sam the Sloth, a blue rose, and a box that says Someone Loves You. Coincidence? A sign?

Much the same way I investigated the playlist of music on YouTube when I heard three magical songs played nearly in succession at the nail salon, I went to the website selling these cute gifts. I wanted to see how many types of critters they had so that I knew the odds of seeing the sloth. If they had only three stuffed critters, then it wouldn't be such a big deal. But it turns out they have over forty adorable critters, and the one that came up in my ad was a sloth. Sam the Sloth.

After my session with Mandy, I pulled out onto the highway. If I'd been three seconds earlier, I would have been able to sweep in front of all the cars that had just been released by the traffic light. But that wasn't the case. There was a steady flow coming at me, and I could see I'd be sitting awhile. While I sat waiting to safely pull into traffic, I thought of those times when something tragic happens and you wonder whether a second or two would have made a difference. When you're in a car accident, for instance, even if it's just a fender bender, you often wonder whether you could have avoided it if you had just missed that light or made that light and not been in that exact moment at that exact time. Or if one tiny detail of your day had been different, like maybe you let someone pull out in front of you or you chatted with a stranger in the parking lot or offered to put their shopping cart back for them, how many times in that day would you have avoided an accident and never known it?

When Piper was killed chasing a cat on February 21, 2016, it was a Sunday night. Sundays at the beach in February are very quiet times. Generally I could probably walk down the middle of the street for several minutes before a car would come my way. But on the night Piper was killed, a cat she was chasing darted across the street. Piper followed after, running like a gazelle. I knew if she was running at full throttle she could cross the road in about two seconds. Nevertheless, at that exact moment, and with no one else around, she crossed the road at the *exact* second the car came. One second sooner and the cat would have been hit. One second later and Piper would have lived that night.

Being that her death came at such a low point in my life, I wondered at the time what purpose there could have been behind this tragedy. I was furious with God. That's the day I shouted to Him, "You don't come to my house and I won't come to yours!" I could not comprehend why God would take away the only thing I loved. Dave and I were separated at that time, and Piper was all I had.

Years later, this came up in conversation with Mandy. She suggested the possibility that if Piper hadn't died, I may never have reunited with Dave. She was right. About two weeks after Piper died, I went to visit Dave in Florida. If there was anyone who could have helped me through my grief, it was Dave. That was the opening of our communication. If Piper hadn't died that night, I may never have had a reason to visit Dave. Imagine where our lives would have ended up if we hadn't reunited. It was because of our time apart and the work we did on our marriage when Dave returned that we were able to create a more solid connection. Even Bobby suggested that our marriage was strengthened by our time apart and that marriages often don't survive catastrophic events like cancer.

Was that God working in mysterious ways? Or was it just an unfortunate event followed by a fortunate event?

When is enough evidence enough evidence?

49

Tuesday, January 23

*L*ife is so different now. I can't imagine where my mind will be in a year or five. I suppose I'm "settling in."

This past Sunday was the twelve-week anniversary of Dave's death. I started sorting through his personal belongings that day. Everything except his clothing. When Dave and I married, he moved into my house and brought along a dozen or so plastic totes. No furniture, just his clothes and totes. For years he joked that everything he owned was in those few bins and all the rest of the stuff in the house was mine. Inside many of those bins were things he was holding onto for his kids while they were going off to college. Being that I have an aversion to too much clutter, I chimed in to suggest that once the kids bought a house, it would be time for them to take their bins. He agreed that was reasonable, so the number of totes we stored whittled down as the years passed.

We went through all of Dave's "keep-it bins" together the month before he died. Of all the sentimental possessions I found, including the itinerary and all the paperwork from our trip to Hawaii nearly twenty-three years earlier, my favorite object was a little clay bowl Dave made when he was about five years old. Initially, I triple-wrapped it in bubble wrap and put it back in the bin so it wouldn't get broken. But items like this are meant to be enjoyed, so on Sunday I moved it to the curio for display. My hope is that when our grandsons are dads and grandpas, they will look at this little bowl and remember their grandpa was once a little boy.

As I sorted through Dave's closet, I made small piles for family members. Each of Dave's kids as well as each grandson will get one. Everything left got repacked and consolidated into the bins. Now there are only four bins left. I find it somewhat incredible that someone's life can be encapsulated inside four bins.

I finally moved Dave's computer off the dining table. It's been in the exact same place since he died. I don't know whether I'll look at that empty chair to talk to him now. I feel like his image is already getting fuzzy in the three places he usually sat. But I often envision us "pinballing" down the hallway together arm-in-arm, and I spend lots of time thinking of Dave before he got sick . . . just like he wanted me to do.

Dave is pretty much always in my head. It's not a conscious thought, he's just always there. Some days there are bouts of crying followed by more crying followed by hard sobbing. And some days there's just sadness.

I've been through many difficult times in my fifty-nine years. Usually it's due to circumstances that will change and need to be "toughed out." That's one of the thoughts that gets most of us through the tough times: Things change. But this is permanent. The only thing that will change is my adaptation to my new circumstances.

I'm getting better at filling my days with distractions. My quest for God is ongoing, but I'm being swayed that He does exist in some form. I prayed the other day about something very specific, something very unlikely to happen. It actually did happen, but it's too personal to put into words. Suffice to say, I continue to be in awe that God could actually be real. I see no negative side to believing in God even if I'm being fooled. I think living a life following the Golden Rule can only make the world a better place.

Still, I'm stuck in neutral believing that I will never see Dave again. The thought of that is really unbearable for me. I suppose even if there is some kind of eternal life, it won't be the kind of reunion I'd like to imagine. If it were, what would happen to spouses that have lost two husbands or wives they loved dearly? Although, the idea of being greeted at the pearly gates by all the dogs I've ever loved is quite comforting.

Love is the message of God I continue to find—love for people, love for animals, love for nature. Love for animals and nature comes quite naturally to me. I'm working on love for people. I'm so fortunate . . . or blessed . . . to have the love of many people around me. They show that love by checking in with me through random texts and inviting me for dinner, coffee, or a walk on the beach. I'm working on sending that love back in the direction of others.

I spoke to Mum last night. Again she said, "You've got a lot of love to give." It reminded me of that night Dave said, "You deserve a lot of love."

It looks like it really does work both ways.

Wednesday, January 24

What a difference a day makes! Today was pivotal. That's the funny thing about significant days. No one says, "Today something incredible will happen" or "I will have an epiphany today." It doesn't happen like that, just like people don't say, "Today I will have a fatal embolism."

The day started out with coffee and the morning news, just like every other day. In the usual way, I said good morning to Dave as soon as my eyes opened and then sat in bed with coffee and my laptop. But after my morning two cups of coffee, before my feet hit the floor for the day, I decided to pray. Molly is having very important scans tomorrow at the same place Dave had scans for three years. I wanted to pray for her, and I wanted to pray for two other friends who have some medical stuff going on. I usually ask God to make Himself a part of my day and to help me down a path that eases my pain. I had a lot to ask for this morning, and I wanted to do it all before the day got going.

You would think if something pivotal were going to happen it would mean I had a spiritual awakening, or at the very least been besieged by blue butterflies. But life-changing events can happen in the most inconsequential ways.

The morning buzzed along uneventfully until I got a text from one of Dave's air force buddies. I haven't seen him since the weekend of the funeral and he was checking on me. In his message he wrote, "Stay strong. David always told me you were the strongest person he knew." Something happened to me when I read that. We all love to hear nice things our spouses have said about us out of earshot, but this really hit home. Many people have told me I'm strong, and I know I'm strong. But hearing that Dave, my person I have such respect and admiration for, said this to someone else with no intention of it getting back to me left me speechless. Suddenly I felt incredibly resilient. If anything, Dave's conviction in me is what's going to lead me to believe I can survive this.

Oddly enough, after this text I got four other signs that Dave is working hard from the other side to send comfort to those who love him. This continues to reinforce in my mind that we need people. God is about relationships. He wants us to love others and have healthy relationships. If it weren't for the relationships I have with Cathy, Megan, and Dave's air force buddy, I wouldn't have known about all the other signs.

My belief in God is strengthening. As much as I'd like to have an "aha" moment when I suddenly have strong convictions that God and the afterlife exist, I don't believe that's the way faith happens. I think it develops over time. And I think it happens just the way it's happening now: through praying, loving, and accepting the love of those around me.

Tonight, instead of my usual shot of rock and bourbon, I opted for a glass of wine. Somehow it seemed a cocktail that was more celebratory than grief-numbing was in order.

50

Friday, January 26

While Dave and I lived together for nearly twenty-two years, his words were always able to comfort me. For many years before we were married, when I would show up at his office in my professional capacity, Dave made me feel like the only one in the room. Seven years later when we went to Hawaii, he was still able to make me feel that way. And nearly thirty years after I met him, he continued to share his magic with me. He made me feel important in his life. He comforted and calmed me like no one else. And he cared for me and put my interests before his. Even though his physical being is no longer here, his words sent to me through his air force buddy continue to comfort me.

I've had a couple of shoulder surgeries over the years. The most recent one was pretty invasive and was expected to be followed by intense rehabilitation. I don't really remember the pain after the surgery. Much the way a woman experiences childbirth—she knows she had contractions and pushed the equivalent of a bowling bowl out of her lady parts, but she can't remember what the pain felt like   that's how it was with my shoulder surgery, and any other surgery I've had for that matter. I remember needing Dave to help me change clothes and cook meals for a few days, but I can't remember what the pain felt like. I should remember, though, because it was many, many months before I could raise my arm over my head.

But when I think of the day Dave took his final breath, his last twenty-four hours, or even his final two weeks, I not only *remember* everything that happened but can still *feel* it. I can feel the pain. I can feel the loss. I don't just remember how it felt, I actually feel it.

I don't have any regrets about that. There's a price for this kind of love. It's the kind where love leaks out of your eyes and we call it tears, the kind where you know you're a better person for having known and loved the one you lost, the kind where you forge ahead not because of your love of life but because the one you lost loved you so much it would devastate him to see you not love yourself.

I can see I'm taking baby steps in the direction of healing. I've started listening to music in the car again, although I'm still selective and avoid most songs that will really set me off on a crying jag. Sometimes at night I listen to "Nine Minutes of Tears." I play it when I actually want to cry.

The other night I decided to take a bath, and I climbed into the tub the "right" way. I sat facing the way I used to sit before the nights of Tub Talks. As I sat there, I spoke to Dave as I do throughout the day: "Dave, look how I'm sitting in the tub. This feels wrong. I think I need to sit the other way so I can imagine you with me." Knowing Dave as I do, I instinctively recited the words he would have chosen if he were physically standing beside me: "Baby, I'm right next to you no matter which way you sit in the damn tub." I smiled knowing that's true. I spun around 180 degrees before I was done, just so I could visualize his face, his head resting back on the rubber pillow, his eyes closed. I'm going to allow myself that pleasure as often as I'd like.

I'm now sure that this God journey is what will help ease my pain. When I started my research, I certainly wanted to believe. If nothing else, it's bothered me for years that I can't commit one way or the other. God versus no God. I just hate living in the gray! As the weeks have passed, I've felt closer and closer to whomever this almighty power is.

Yesterday I prayed hard again for Molly. Months after radiation and chemotherapy, she finally had her scans. Depending on the results of this imaging, she could be looking at a life-changing surgery. I was the third person she called after getting the results. "There is no sign of disease," she said. Just incredible! For now, she can live her life cancer free. I don't know that God had something to do with that, but *when is enough evidence enough evidence?*

There's no doubt the one truth uncovered in my search for God is that people need people. I thought without Dave I would pull away from everyone. Nothing could be further from the truth. The bottomless heart full of love I had for Dave didn't die with him. I still have it. He set such a good example of how to love others in his own special way. Of course, I still love my Dave as my end-all and be-all, but all the love in me needs to be shared with those around me.

I'll be taking some trips with the camper in the next few months. Next month will be the rip-the-bandage-off trip. The following month, Teddy and I will spend nearly a week in Georgia. Maybe having someone else in the camper with me will help make it bearable. And I finally started planning a trip for August. I don't have all the details ironed out, but I do have two weeks booked in a state park in Kansas. I'll be volunteering at an equine rescue and rehabilitation facility. After that, I might just go where the wind blows me.

Oh, and I stopped by the tattoo parlor yesterday, the one where I got the tattoo on my left ankle. Up until now, that tattoo has symbolized me completely. My life's purpose, or so I thought, was about loving dogs, rescuing dogs, training dogs . . . all things dog-related. There's a reason Dave said he wanted to come back as my dog. Anyway, I spoke to the tattoo artist about a blue butterfly tattoo. Remembering Dave was not a fan of tattoos and the discussion about a butterfly tattoo after he passed, I could hear him chuckling and saying, "Sure. I sent you all kinds of signs yesterday and now you go and get a tattoo. Go for it, Snooks. Do whatever makes you happy."

Saturday, January 28

I now have a beautiful blue butterfly tattooed on the inside of my left forearm. She has a shadow next to her, so it looks like she's gently fluttering down my arm. I wanted it in a place where everyone would see it. I want everyone to know about the blue butterfly and what it means to me. It means there is something more. It means there is something after this. It means Dave is still with me.

I don't know whether God is really here, but I do know there's something bigger than what we know waiting for us. After all, *when is enough evidence enough evidence?* I asked Dave to continue to send me blue butterflies . . . they make me so happy.

51

Sunday, January 29

*D*ave died thirteen weeks ago today.

I've been watching Pastor Bobby online the last couple of Sundays and thinking all week about actually going to church today. There are four morning services, and the middle two are the most crowded, but I went to the second one anyway. As I walked out of the house, I asked Dave to come to church with me, and I prayed: *Please God, give me the courage to do this. I know I shouldn't be afraid to go to church, but it's going to be so hard without Dave.*

I pulled up to the building a little early. The last time I was there was for Dave's memorial service, and I'd been wearing a dress covered in images of butterflies. I decided to leave my phone in the car. I'm never without my phone, a habit more ingrained when I knew there was a possibility Dave might need me. After all, what could happen that I'd need a phone for in the next forty-five minutes?

When I entered the lobby, I saw Bobby. It was between services and he was making rounds talking to the congregation. On a Sunday, when you catch Bobby at church, it's like he's dumped a pot of caffeine down his gullet. He gets really amped up talking about Jesus. Clearly, Jesus is his drug of choice. He casually escorted the people in front of me down the hall to the pews; I figured they must be new to the church. Then he saw me. His face lit up. He wrapped his arms around me and hugged me like he hadn't seen me in a decade. He knows the path I've been on, and my being there means my faith is deepening. He didn't have to say any words; he exuded excitement!

Dave and I didn't attend church regularly, but when we did we always took the same two seats. I contemplated sitting someplace new, but I wanted the comfort of familiarity. I sat in the exact seat I always took, leaving the two on my left empty. The church filled up quickly, and a married couple took the two empty seats. I smiled and said hello. In all honesty, if I'm not sitting next to someone I know, I prefer to have empty seats beside me, but that was unlikely during this busy service.

At the beginning of the service, the band played and we all stood and sang. As I scanned the room, I noticed a woman who was located two rows in front of me. She was in my direct line of sight and about five or six feet away. I was completely dazzled. Although just an ordinary-looking woman wearing jeans, she was wearing a white top covered with blue butterflies with just a few orange ones thrown in. I looked up and smiled. I knew Dave was there. I knew he was with me. And I was kicking myself that I didn't have my phone to take a picture of this incredible shirt bedazzled with butterflies.

Eventually we sat, and Bobby spoke for a spell before encouraging us all to "love up on one another." I think that phrase is pretty much a Southern thing. Being a Northerner, I never heard it, but I've started using it since I moved here. I introduced myself to the couple sitting to my left, and we made a bit of small talk. They told me they usually come to the first service but for some reason they had come to this one today. We settled down for Bobby's sermon.

After Bobby was done preaching, he told us to stand for another song. I asked the woman to my left if she would do me a favor: "Can you take a picture of that woman's shirt, and I'll give you my number to text it to me?"

She looked a little puzzled, maybe a little suspicious, so I rolled my arm over so she could see my beautiful new tattoo. "The blue butterfly is significant to me," I said.

When she saw the tattoo, she nodded and looked for her phone. That's when I blurted out, "My husband died thirteen weeks ago today and I asked him to send me blue butterflies to comfort me."

She had a rush of emotion, so much so that her husband quickly turned his head to see what was taking place between us. We both started to cry and hug. I was thinking about the things I've learned these last thirteen weeks about leaning on people . . . loving . . . having relationships.

She took the picture as we stood for a song, then set her phone down for me to enter my number after the service. As we stood side by side with our hands resting on the row in front of us, I felt the urge to take her hand. I set my hand atop hers, and she returned my grasp. I could hear her still recovering from the startling news I dumped on her and wondered if maybe I was put there for her, for what's going on in her life. She wasn't supposed to be at this service . . . I always have my phone on me . . . her and her husband happened to take the two empty seats next to me . . . *When is enough evidence enough evidence?*

When the service was over, she asked if I had any plans. I told her Nora is coming over to collect a bunch of Dave's shirts to make me a memory blanket and pillows for family and then we're going to lunch. The woman seemed pleased I had plans.

When I got back to my car, I saw her text: "God is with you and so is your husband."

52

Friday, March 22

$\mathcal{I}$ had every intention of ending this journal after seeing the butterfly shirt in church. It seemed like I was on an upward trajectory. What could go wrong?

I've heard the phrase "Grief is not linear," and I've seen that to be true. Good days have hard moments. Hard days have good moments. A crying jag is always waiting around the corner.

I just noticed today that it's been about six months since I started this journal. Six months ago, I never imagined Dave's death wouldn't be the peaceful death I hoped for but instead far worse than everything I feared.

On February 6, day one hundred following Dave's death (for those of you without OCD that's fourteen weeks and two days), I really tanked. I tend to be very aware of dates and anniversaries, which probably isn't a surprise since I'm still counting the anniversary of his death in weeks—this coming Sunday is twenty-one weeks. That morning I sent a text to Patrick and Margaret: "100 days. To the rest of the world today is Tuesday, February 6. To me it is 100 days." Patrick's reply was sensible and comforting: "Tomorrow will be 101 days. He's watching you."

It was also the day I heard on the news that Toby Keith died. He was sixty-two years old and fought stomach cancer for eighteen months. Various news outlets mentioned the phrase,

"He passed away peacefully, surrounded by his family." That's the biggest crock of bullshit. Nobody dies peacefully from cancer, unless they go into a coma. Every time I hear that phrase it makes me crazy. When I saw his wife, who was his advocate and caregiver, standing at one of his concerts, she reminded me of me. I completely lost it. I felt so bad for her. Thinking of the cancer train they rode for eighteen months caused me to relive the past three years. I spiraled downward for days and days. Okay, actually, I spiraled for weeks.

About two weeks later I had my first panic attack. I felt it building all day and just kept putting it off. Finally, it hit. Finding my breathing so out of control was scary. I managed to regain my composure on my own, but I resolved myself to the idea that I might need medication to get through this.

So at my next appointment with Mandy, I asked for her thoughts regarding medication. She thought it might be helpful to curb my OCD thoughts just a tad, take the edge off the anxiety, and get my body used to functioning with a bit more serotonin. I consider it a personal challenge not to have to add "maintenance meds" as I trudge into my aging years, but I also pride myself on my problem-solving ability, and it seemed like this would be a good tool to add to my toolbox. I started on the meds about a month ago, and I do feel better. I don't know whether my improvement is the natural progression of grief or the daily pill, but there haven't been any ill side effects, and I'm sure I won't stay on these forever.

I had the virtual appointment with the psychic medium. I think it was a complete fail. There was nothing he said worth convincing me that he was communicating with any of my loved ones who have passed. It really infuriates me that people make a living off other people's grief and desperation. There was only one detail that stood out as noteworthy: As soon as we began our session, I observed his well-decorated office background and noticed that hanging on the wall behind him was a picture of a blue butterfly. How odd, right?

I spent a few days in the camper alone, ripping off the bandage. I was right. It was awful. I spoke to Dave for nearly three days straight. I also journaled often. This was my entry on day one of the short trip:

> I slept horribly last night. I was constantly too hot, yet the heater was set to only 61°F. I've gotten used to sprawling out in our king-size bed at home; I have half that in the camper.
>
> My morning camper routine was always quietly getting my coffee, cranking the heat up for Dave, and moving back to my bed with my Mac. Usually Sadie would join me on the bed at this point. Dave would continue sleeping. Except now he's not here. I look at his empty bed, all made up with the pillows still perfect, and I can't imagine how he's not here.
>
> I remember one of our trips when I texted with my friend David one morning. I told him I was watching Dave sleep and couldn't imagine one day he wouldn't be here; I just couldn't imagine it. That day has come and I still can't believe it.
>
> I can see now why I couldn't imagine it. It's like trying to see yourself sitting on a cloud. All you think about is what it would feel like to be sitting on a puffy, white, cottony cloud, dangling your feet over the edge like in a childhood cartoon. You don't think about how strong the winds would be at that altitude. You don't think about the icy cold temperature. You don't think about falling from the sky. You just think about what's right in front of you . . . the obvious.

That's what happens when you try to imagine your person being gone forever while he's still here. You imagine his death. You imagine his absence. You imagine what it means for him not to be present to talk to, to hold, to be held by. But you don't think about all the other abstract things until they happen.

You don't realize you will replay every moment of your life with him, second-guessing yourself and wondering all the time whether he realized you loved him as much as you could at the time, that you wish you could do it all over again. You remember the time he said to you, "No one has ever loved me totally and completely," and you wish you never made him feel that way.

You know in your heart that over the years you made up for lost time by loving him unconditionally, and at the end of his life he knew he was loved totally and completely by you. But you still constantly find fault with yourself. You berate yourself for not realizing how lucky you were in your life—not just for being married to the man who changed your life for the better but for other aspects as well, such as having a great job, enough money, good friends, and friends and family who are healthy.

You don't realize that even though you knew his life would end due to cancer, you really can't wrap your head around him being gone forever after it happens. You think if you could see him and talk to him for one hour, even twenty years from now, that would give you the hope you need to keep going. But you know that can't happen.

Still, you try to negotiate with God. You lean into God. You ask Him for help and to be present in your life. You believe that if you can believe in God, you can believe your person is somehow okay.

The idea of him not existing . . . not being . . . just panics you. Circle back to God. You ask Him why he's not helping you. You pray, you get down on your knees, you beg for help, yet you don't feel He hears you. You think back to your deep dive to discover whether God is real. When is enough evidence enough evidence?

You're always looking for a blue butterfly. And when you hear a song on the radio that makes you think of him, you wonder whether that's a sign or a coincidence. If you're wired like me, it has to be more than one song to believe it's a sign.

You don't realize you'll feel you're on a hamster wheel. The only break is when you go to sleep, and even that isn't a break sometimes. Even when it is, everything picks up right when you get up in the morning.

It. Never. Stops.

Round and round.

The grief. The sorrow. The continuing sadness and emptiness. Forever.

You didn't realize that when he died, the color would leave your world.

You didn't realize that hope would die with him.

When I made the drive home after an emotionally exhausting three days, I drove the exact same route home that I drove on the way to the campground. Oddly enough, I saw not one, not two, but four of those blue butterfly yard signs that say, "Pray for Insley." How could I have missed all four of these on my way to the campsite? Is it possible they were just put out over the weekend? On four different properties?

Two weeks later, I spent time with Teddy camping in that state park in Georgia. We actually had a lot of fun! Certainly the first fun I've had since before Dave died. We covered about twenty-one miles in three days, hiking in the woods and wandering around the campground. This gave us lots of time for conversation. Considering this bright, young man rarely stops talking, we covered many subjects. One of my favorites went like this:

> Teddy: "I'm really funny. That's why all the girls like me. I get my sense of humor from Grandpa."
>
> Me: "Yes, Teddy, you do. That's definitely how Grandpa got all the ladies."
>
> Teddy: "I get my good looks from Grandpa too."
>
> Me: "Yes, Teddy, you most definitely do."

I'm still working on planning a trip in August. I'm having difficulty finding activities along the way to my destination that won't magnify Dave's absence. I think in time planning trips will get easier. But for now it's a challenge.

Being a staunch believer in self-help, I still see Mandy regularly, and I've also added in a grief counselor. I just started with him, but I figure it can't hurt.

There's more to the grieving process than grieving the loss of Dave. I grieve for the person I was. I grieve for my old life. As imperfect as it was, it was my life and I got quite used to it. Now, besides feeling that grief, I feel guilty that I didn't appreciate my old life. I mean, when does this shit stop?

My relationship with my mother has been surprisingly healthy. She filters her words, she apologizes if she thinks she said something inappropriate, and I actually initiate conversation with her since she's been more pleasant. I wish this change could have happened forty years ago. Dave would be happy to witness our blossoming relationship. I guess it's never too late to change if someone wants to put in the effort, but I'm still cautious to protect myself.

I go to the cemetery about every other week. After my first couple of visits, I decided I want to bring Dave a little something when I visit. He loved Payday candy bars. Whenever he'd buy one at a convenience store, he'd get back in the car, peel off the end of the wrapper, and offer me a bite. I usually took one bite and gave the rest back to him. So I bought a bag of fun-size Payday bars. Every time I go to the cemetery, I bring one with me. I tear off the wrapper, take a bite, and place the rest on his headstone.

Megan visited me without the kids right before I took Teddy camping. I asked her if she'd like to go to the cemetery with me. I brought two Payday bars and shared my new tradition with her. If you're familiar with Payday bars, you know they're loaded with peanuts. We joked that during one of these visits, I'm going to find a family of squirrels hanging around Dave's grave, waiting for these mysteriously appearing candy bars.

Not far from the cemetery is one of the rage rooms I looked into. I asked Megan if she'd like to go with me. I think she knew I needed to beat the crap out of something. I'm not going to say that swinging a baseball bat helped me alleviate any long-term anger, but I will say the vacuum cleaner that was in the room was unrecognizable by the time we left.

I'm still reading far more than I used to, but I wouldn't say I've been a voracious reader lately. I'm not on the constant hunt for answers, as I realize now that answers don't exist for some questions. I realize it, but it doesn't make it any easier for me to accept.

I'm reading a book in which the author describes herself as having a metaphysical crisis when she was nine years old. She writes, "Soon I would be a teenager, then middle-aged, then elderly, then dead."[12] She went on to describe how some of us are hardwired for anxiety about mortality, some of us are indifferent and acknowledge the inevitable, and some of us downright embrace the idea. I was rather happy to see there's at least one other person in the world who's been struggling with the idea of death since childhood. Oh yeah, apparently it's linked to "control issues." Go figure.

Today I went to the gym, and as I was leaving it occurred to me that I hadn't thought about Dave the entire time I was there. On the drive home, I stopped for some groceries. As I wandered the aisles reading nutrition labels on new products, like I have for the last thirty years, I realized how normal it felt to be doing that. Then the music playing in the store switched to something that struck a chord in me, and I started feeling guilty that I thought of Dave only on and off today. He's always in my heart, and he's always on my mind, but it's not always as a conscious thought. I'm sure the guilt is natural, and I imagine it's actually a sign that I'm headed in the direction of healing.

I've slowed down my alcohol consumption, and I haven't played "Nine Minutes of Tears" in weeks. At least once a day, I still cry like it's October 29. I just find it mind-numbing that he isn't here. I don't know why that's so baffling to me.

I haven't missed an opportunity to write messages to Dave on the steamy shower wall, but they've become more elaborate. Sometimes rather than just "I love you" or "I miss you," I write an entire paragraph. I say good morning and good night to Dave daily and tell him I love him and miss him. I would give ten years off my life to have him back for a day, as long as he wasn't in pain.

Sloth sleeps with me every night and travels with me on every camping trip. He gives me a chuckle nearly every morning. When I make the bed, Sloth is usually nestled somewhere under the covers. After the quilt is straight and smooth, I often notice a lump. Realizing it's Sloth once again, I smile while reaching under the blankets to drag him out of the bed. Hiding under the covers is such a Dave-like thing to do. He loved to sleep, so it's no surprise his spirit animal does the same.

I dream of Dave regularly, often a version that goes something like this:

> *Dave and I are together in our normal life. He looks healthy. He has a work thing to do, some sort of convention. He's in work mode, wearing his button-down blue shirt and his sleeves rolled up just past his Popeye-like forearms but below the elbows, the way I like it.*
>
> *He's busy inside the building. I've been outside on a ladder. It occurs to me that I have an opportunity to tell him all the things I should have. I climb down the ladder, walk inside, and watch him delegate. I think to myself, "Now I can tell him how I've loved being married to the guy who's the boss. He's so impressive when he works—so smart, so sharp—I can tell him how he's the best thing that ever happened to me and what a great husband he is."*
>
> *But as I have this thought, I wonder why I know to tell him this now. Why didn't I know to say these things before? There must have been a catalyst that made me think to tell him these things now.*
>
> *And just like that, I remember he died. He died and that's why I know I need to tell him these things. And with that, he simply evaporates.*

That seems to be the theme of my dreams. And I usually remember Dave died before I wake up. When I do wake up after a dream like that, I say, "Good morning, Dave. That was a rough one."

I had at least a half dozen dreams that resembled that sequence of events until I finally had one in which I knew he was dead, but I sat next to him anyway, wrapped my arms around him, and told him he was the greatest husband ever and I love him dearly. I guess my brain worked out what it needed to, because that was the last time I had that type of dream.

Gradually, my guilt over not loving Dave hard enough during the early years is subsiding as I'm realizing I was incapable at that time. It's *because* of the first thirteen years of our marriage that I was able to move on to the latter part. It's *because* Dave loved and trusted me completely that I learned to love and trust. Dave healed some very old scars.

I can honestly say that I'm not suffering the way I was a month or two ago. Nothing about this is easy, though. I still share my grief with friends and family, but you can't walk around like a wet rag day after day and expect people to tolerate being around you. What people see on the outside is certainly not what's going on inside. I'm like the duck analogy: I'm looking carefree as I glide across the pond, but below I'm treading furiously.

Being proactive in my self-care has been helpful; it probably gives me the sense of control I crave. Love has helped me too—my love for others and their love for me.

I wonder all the time whether Dave can see me. My gut tells me he can't, but of course I don't know for sure. I think it really comes down to making a choice whether to believe or not believe in what happens after we die. Are we over-over, or is there an afterlife? Unfortunately, I think my inability to choose to believe is an OCD thing. I think somehow it's linked to having issues with control, certainty, and perfection.

If Dave can see me now, I'm sure my sadness causes him sorrow, no different from when he was here with me. Conversely, when I'm riding a horse, petting a dog, rescuing a bird, talking to Megan, or hooking up the camper, he's smiling happily, nodding that he knew I was strong enough to navigate his death.

I certainly don't know whether my soul will be over-over when I die, but I am sure of one thing: If death doesn't mean over-over when I close my eyes for the last time, I will be welcomed to the other side by a warm hug. Behind that hug will be my Bumpy with his beautiful blue eyes and jolly smile. With a smirk on his face he'll say, "I've been waiting for you, Snooks. You're gonna love it here!"

THE END

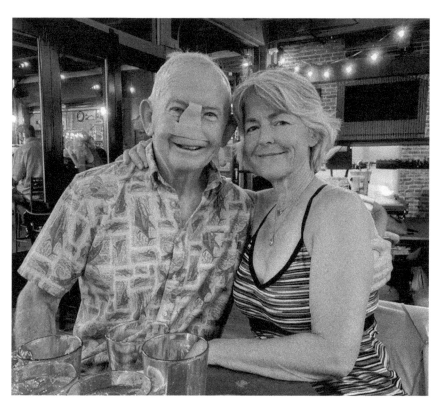

July 28, 2023: BLT 2023, my Dave and me

A Couple More Things

Unless someone like you cares a whole awful lot, nothing is going to get better. It's not.

~Dr. Seuss

I am confident you will walk away from my book knowing you read a love story. I believe you will also realize that should you ever find yourself in my position, you *will* be able to manage your new life. Very. Slowly. It takes a lot of time and grace with yourself and a tremendous number of tears. One breath. One moment. One day. One foot in front of the other.

With over 2,500 women becoming widows every day in this country, the likelihood that you know a woman who has lost her husband is high. Few people know what to do for a recent widow, especially when she says she doesn't need anything. Here's my best advice:

 Send her messages reminding her how much you care, but don't expect a response.

 Send her heart emojis with statements, not questions. Words like, "I'm thinking of you," "You are often on my mind and always in my heart," or simply "I love you" provide comfort.

 If you think this book would be helpful to her, gift her a copy.

Unless you're very close, don't bother asking her, "How are you?" That puts too much pressure on her to come up with something positive.

 Find out what time of day is most difficult for her, and contact her then. Mine was the dinner hour; that was when I most needed to communicate with someone. But I never wanted to bother anyone during dinner, so I'd end up spending time with Captain Morgan, Malibu, or my good friend Mr. Bourbon to make those one to two hours pass less painfully.

There are two important issues related to cancer that I'd like to make sure I convey to you before you go:

1. I wish I had known the benefits of palliative care years sooner than I did. I believed it was another word for hospice, essentially end-of-life care. It's not. Palliative care is specialized medical care for people living with a serious illness such as cancer, heart failure, dementia, Parkinson's disease, and Lou Gehrig's disease. Patients may receive palliative care to manage the symptoms of their disease soon after its diagnosis. It can be complementary to the treatment they're receiving to treat their serious illness but is not a substitute for treatment or your specialist's care. It's meant to enhance a patient's quality of life whether their disease is terminal or not. And palliative care is covered by Medicare and most private insurance.

If you find yourself or your loved one being diagnosed with a serious illness and dealing with unmanageable symptoms, palliative care may be right for you. Please ask your medical team about it. Even if it's not the right course of treatment for you or your loved one now, it may be in the future, and your provider may actually be glad to learn you're open to it. Until we redefine the current understanding of palliative care, your provider may be uneasy to initiate the idea for fear of losing your confidence. Be your own advocate!

2. Although sinonasal cancers are extremely rare, each year approximately 3,000 people in the United States are diagnosed with them. Men are at twice the risk of women, and most of them are between the ages of fifty and seventy. Because they are rare cancers, they don't receive the amount of funding for clinical trials and research that many of the other more common cancers receive; therefore, the treatment doesn't change much from year to year and the survival rate shows minimal improvement.

The daily pill that helped stabilize Dave's cancer during his last year is considered a targeted therapy. It's currently being marketed as a drug for thyroid, kidney, liver, and endometrial cancer, but not for sinonasal cancer. With more funding and more research, protocols can be developed that are specifically designed to treat sinonasal and paranasal cancers. In turn, this will improve the chances of survival for those facing these rare diseases.

In memory of Dave, I am donating a share of the proceeds from the sale of this book to the Skull Base Surgery Fund at the University of North Carolina (UNC) in Chapel Hill. Gifts to the fund will be used to support clinical, research, and education initiatives focused on skull base and sinonasal cancers within the Department of Otolaryngology/Head & Neck Surgery at UNC Health.

If our story has touched you and you want to help make a difference in the world, I ask you to make a donation in Dave's name to the UNC Health Foundation Fund.

Direct Link:
https://give.unc.edu/hfdonate?p=GLIB

Those who would like to donate by check can do so by addressing the check to "UNC Health Foundation." Please include "In memory of David J. Gilbride – #349426" in the memo line. Your check can be mailed to:

UNC Health Foundation
123 W. Franklin St., Suite 510
Chapel Hill, NC 27516

If you would like to contact me, I'd love to hear from you! I can be reached at TheBlueButterflyInMe@gmail.com.

Notes

1. Henry Scott Holland, "The Ship," All Poetry, accessed June 5, 2024, https://allpoetry.com/poem/13603447-The-Ship-by-Henry-Scott-Holland.

2. *Shall We Dance?*, directed by Peter Chelsom (2004; New York, NY: Miramax, 2005), DVD.

3. C. S. Lewis, *Mere Christianity* (Touchstone, 1996), 175–176.

4. NCI Staff, "Heart Attack, Stroke Risk May Be Elevated Following Cancer Diagnosis," National Cancer Institute, August 25, 2017, https://www.cancer.gov/news-events/cancer-currents-blog/2017/heart-attack-stroke-risk-cancer.

5. *It's a Wonderful Life*, directed by Frank Capra (1946; New York, NY: RKO Radio Pictures, 2001), DVD.

6. Lynne Eldridge, "What Is Anticipatory Grief?," Verywell Health, last modified July 15, 2023, https://www.verywellhealth.com/understanding-anticipatory-grief-and-symptoms-2248855#:~:text.

7. Jeannie MacDonald, "Classic Hollywood: Classic Couples: James & Gloria Stewart," The Music Hall, December 15, 2022, https://www.themusichall.org/blog/classic-hollywood-classic-couples-james-gloria-stewart/.

8. MacDonald, "Classic Hollywood."

9. C. S. Lewis, "Christian Apologetics," in *God in the Dock*, ed. Walter Hopper (Wm. B. Eerdmans Publishing Co.; reprint edition March 24, 1972), essay 10.

10. Kristen French, "The Afterlife Is in Our Heads," Nautilus, September 28, 2022, https://nautil.us/the-afterlife-is-in-our-heads-240441/.

11. C. S. Lewis, *A Grief Observed* (HarperOne, 2015), 9–10.

12. Elizabeth Gilbert, *Eat, Pray, Love* (Riverhead Books, 2007), 152.

About the Author

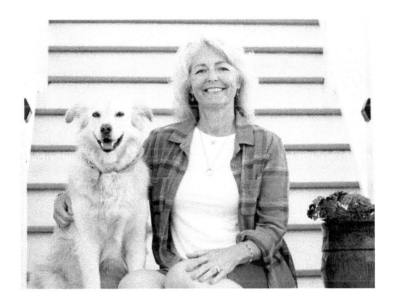

$\mathcal{B}$orn and raised in the suburbs of New Jersey, Patricia Clark was raised as an only child in a single-parent home. At seventeen years old, Patty left home for college, dropping out a year later. She bounced around living in different places and trying different jobs until she decided on a career in law enforcement. She started her career with the Morris County Sheriff's office when she was twenty-five years old.

Over the next ten years, Patty threw herself into her job, homeownership, and her love for her dogs. Spending her free time advocating for animal causes, she has always believed that one person can make a difference; whether it's one plastic bottle recycled or one dog saved from a shelter, one person can impact the world.

Patty met her future husband, David Gilbride, during her work as a sheriff's officer. They lived in New Jersey for thirteen years and retired to Topsail Island, North Carolina, in 2015.

Patty expected her retirement to consist of "doing all the things I didn't have time to do when I was working." Having a strong belief in the importance of volunteerism, she spent the next five years rescuing birds, taking her pet therapy dog to various facilities, and training her rescue dog.

But in 2020 when her husband was diagnosed with a rare, aggressive cancer, she shifted gears to become a full-time advocate and caregiver. For the next three years, Patty and Dave excelled at making memories together that would last her a lifetime. After Dave's death, Patty wrote her first book and discovered her calling was sharing her grief with others. As a critical part of her healing, she realized the topics of death and end-of-life need to become more a part of common conversation. She hopes to encourage people to start talking about these topics with their families so that as a society we can grow more comfortable with the subjects.

Patty is donating much of the proceeds garnered from *Something More Than Love* to the Skull Base Surgery Fund at the University of North Carolina (UNC) in Chapel Hill. Gifts to the fund will be used to support clinical research and education initiatives focused on skull base and sinonasal cancers within the Department of Otolaryngology/Head & Neck Surgery at UNC Health. She hopes to make the cancer journey that she and Dave faced more promising for others.

Patty can be found either on the beaches of Topsail Island, North Carolina, or traveling the country in her camper with her dog.

Donate to the Skull Base Surgery Fund at the University of North Carolina (UNC)

Direct Link:
https://give.unc.edu/hfdonate?p=GLIB

Connect with the Author

Direct Link:
facebook.com/patty.gilbride/

Direct Link:
instagram.com/patty_gilbride_author/